I0555117

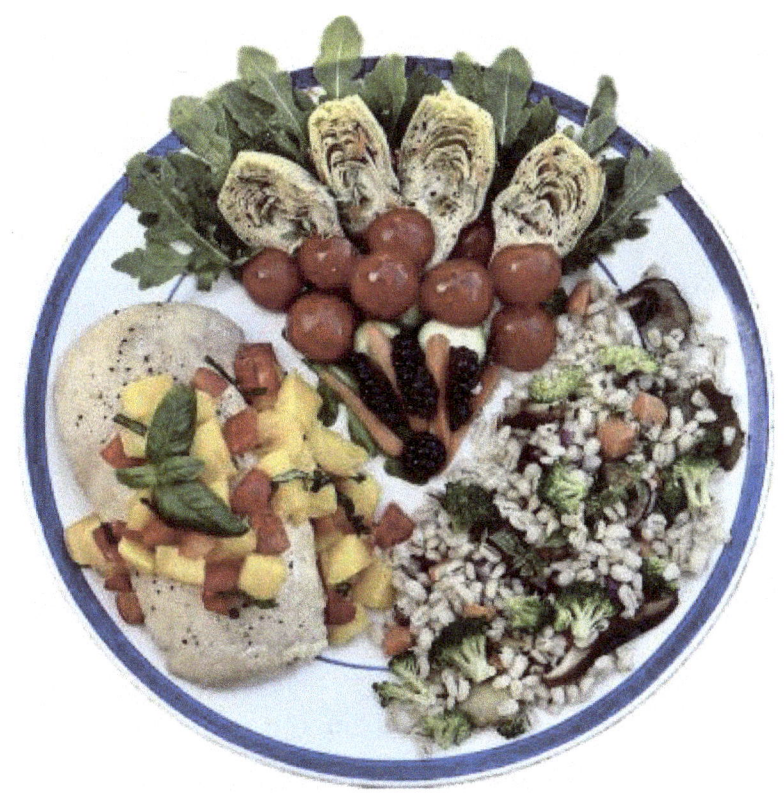

THE
HEALING
PLATE

EAT YOURSELF HEALTHY

DELICIOUS RECIPES TO HELP FIGHT BREAST CANCER

STEPHANY BAUGHMAN

Copyright © 2025, Stephany Baughman

ALL RIGHTS RESERVED

No part of this book may be reproduced or transmitted in any form by any means, electronic or mechanical, including photocopying and recording, or by any information storage and retrieval system,

except as may be expressly permitted in writing from the author.

ISBN:

Published by: Columbus Book Publishers

https://columbusbookpublishers.com/

Printed in the United States of America

Disclaimer:

The information provided in this book, The Healing Plate, is intended for general informational and educational purposes only. It is not intended as a substitute for professional medical advice, diagnosis, or treatment. Always consult your physician or a qualified health care professional before making any changes to your diet, lifestyle, or health care regimen, especially if you have any existing medical conditions, are pregnant, nursing, taking medications, or are under medical supervision.

While the author has made every effort to ensure the accuracy and completeness of the information presented, neither the author nor the publisher assumes any responsibility for errors, omissions, or contrary interpretations of the subject matter. The reader assumes full responsibility for how they choose to use this information.

Statements about the health benefits of foods and recipes included in this book have not been evaluated by the Food and Drug Administration. This book is not intended to diagnose, treat, cure, or prevent any disease.

By using this book, you acknowledge and agree that neither the author nor the publisher shall be held liable for any loss, damage, or injury arising from any information or suggestions contained herein.

Dedication

To My Dad,

You were my greatest cheerleader and my safe place. Losing you far too soon changed me forever, but your love and wisdom guide me still. This book is a tribute to the life you lived and the love you gave so freely. You fought a battle no one should fight, yet your courage and love never wavered. Though you left too soon, your legacy lives on in me and in this work.

"The Lord is close to the brokenhearted and saves those who are crushed in spirit." — Psalm 34:18

Acknowledgments

First and foremost, I want to thank the Lord for leading me to what I didn't even know I was looking for, for opening doors I never thought I'd walk through, and for teaching me how to truly listen—not just to my own thoughts, but to the stories and struggles of others. This book was born from that kind of listening.

To every woman, friend, and client who came to me and said, "I have breast cancer"—thank you. Your honesty, your trust, and your courage opened my eyes and heart in new ways. To those who were starving from treatment and couldn't keep food down, your pain helped me better understand what real nourishment means. So many of the recipes in this book were created for you—and because of you.

To the clients who shared their symptoms, their fears, and their hopes with me—thank you for inspiring me to think beyond prescriptions, to see food as a partner in healing. I believe that great nutrition and thoughtful medicine can work hand in hand, and your journeys helped shape that belief into something practical, compassionate, and real.

To the Health Science Academy, thank you for equipping me with the knowledge and confidence to back up my instincts with science. You gave me the tools I needed to help others with both heart and evidence.

And to my mother—thank you for teaching me how to cook. Not just how to follow a recipe, but how to bring joy, comfort, and flavor to the table. Your love shows up in every dish I make.

This book was never just about food. It's about healing, listening, learning, and loving well. To everyone who has been part of that—this plate is for you.

Foreword

I am honored to introduce this beautifully composed cookbook, in which Stephany has combined her extensive expertise in nutrition and her skills as a chef to write a book designed specifically to support those with breast cancer through their journey. As a surgeon specializing in breast cancer treatment, I have witnessed firsthand the challenges that come with a breast cancer diagnosis—from the profound sense of loss of control and the deep fear of a possibly fatal cancer diagnosis to treatment-related side effects. For most, the treatment process is long and arduous. I also understand the critical importance of nutrition in the healing process. This book is a collection of recipes that are fun to make, crafted to provide not only delicious meals but also to include the essential nutrients needed to support your body during treatment and recovery.

The phrase, "tell me what you eat, and I will tell you who you are," was first attributed to the French gastronome Anthelme Brillat-Savarin in 1825. In his writings, he advocated that the meal process added to life happiness. For me personally, cooking has long been not only how I nurtured myself and my family, but also how I decompressed after long days at work. I enjoyed the process of preparation, especially the chopping, which became a form of mediation, and the final tasting and adjusting of flavors. Cooking can be viewed as a creative, artistic form of self-expression, which also serves the critical function of nurturing our bodies. When you prepare food yourself, you are in control of all the ingredients. You can prioritize fresh, organically farmed produce and humanely raised antibiotic free proteins, avoid processed foods that have been robbed of their nutrients, and you can control portion size. Meals shared with family and friends can provide an opportunity for socialization, which has been demonstrated to improve cancer survival.

Good nutrition during breast cancer isn't about strict rules or perfect meals. It is about listening to your body, focusing on foods that help you feel your best and finding joy in what you eat. From boosting your immune system to managing treatment side effects, the ingredients and cooking methods have been chosen to promote overall well-being. And it's about making mealtimes simple, delicious, and satisfying, even when your appetite, energy levels, or taste preferences change.

Just as no two breast-cancer journeys are the same, there is no one-size-fits-all diet. A healthy diet is not a substitute for critical breast-cancer treatments, such as surgery, anti-estrogens, chemotherapy, or radiation. However, nourishing your body with the right foods can make a significant difference in how you feel and even how well you respond to treatment. Food is also not just fuel, but a form of healing, resilience, and love.

I hope this book serves as a caring companion for you on your journey of healing – one nourishing bite at a time.

Wishing you all the best on your wellness journey,

Daleela Dodge MD

Specialist in Breast Cancer Surgery and in Patient's Health & Wellnes

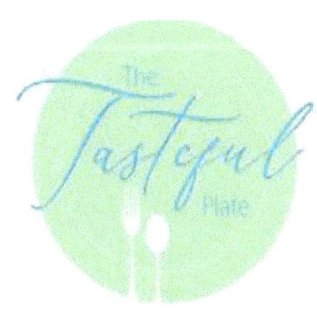

About the Author

Hi, let me introduce myself! My name is Stephany Baughman and I have been passionately helping my clients for over 14 years to achieve better health and vitality. My work has supported people in becoming nutritionally sound, losing weight, going off medications, lowering their A1C, improving sleep, and gaining more energy, just to name a few. More recently, I've expanded my focus to help individuals use food as a powerful tool to combat illnesses within their bodies.

Over the past year, I've had the honor of working alongside physicians, supporting their clients in becoming healthier through mindful, intentional eating. In no way is this intended to take the place of any medications or to diagnose, treat, cure, or prevent disease. Breast cancer, in particular, has touched my life in a deeply personal way through some of my dearest friends. Helping them through their journey inspired me to create this cookbook. My goal is not only to provide delicious recipes but to explain the "why" behind each ingredient so that you can feel confident knowing the food you are eating is actively supporting your body's healing process.

With seven certifications in health and wellness (and currently working on my eighth), I've dedicated my career to empowering others to take charge of their health. Cooking is my passion, and I'm here to show you that healthy food doesn't have to be bland or boring. It can be vibrant, flavorful, and deeply nourishing, both for the body and the soul.

As we walk through this journey together, my heartfelt prayer is that this cookbook will provide more than just recipes; it will offer hope, comfort, and the reassurance that you are feeding your body with love, strength, and healing. Let's savor every bite as we move toward health and wholeness together.

Table of Contents

A Bit About Breast Cancer

According to Pamela Wright, M.D., Medical Director of the Breast Center at Johns Hopkins' Suburban Hospital, Invasive Ductal Carcinoma (IDC), also known as Infiltrating Ductal Carcinoma, is the most common form of breast cancer, accounting for approximately 80% of all breast cancer diagnoses.

Invasive ductal carcinoma occurs when abnormal cells that begin growing in the lining of the milk ducts change and invade the surrounding breast tissue beyond the duct walls. Once these cancer cells breach the duct, they have the potential to spread further. They can enter the lymphatic system or bloodstream, allowing the cancer to travel to other organs and tissues in the body. This spread leads to metastatic breast cancer, which is more challenging to treat.

Another important subtype is HER2-positive breast cancer. This form is characterized by breast cancer cells that have an overexpression of the HER2 receptor, a protein that regulates how breast cells grow, divide, and repair themselves. When too many HER2 receptors are present, breast cells can grow and divide more rapidly than normal, promoting tumor development. HER2-positive cancers tend to be more aggressive but often respond well to targeted therapies such as trastuzumab (Herceptin).

HR refers to hormone receptor status. Tumors that are HR-positive (HR+) have receptors for hormones such as estrogen or progesterone, which can fuel tumor growth. Treatments for HR+ breast cancer often involve hormone-blocking therapies.

HER2 stands for Human Epidermal Growth Factor Receptor 2. Tumors that are HER2-positive (HER2+) produce high levels of the HER2/neu protein, which is associated with more aggressive tumor behavior.

Chemotherapy remains a critical treatment modality but while it targets cancer cells, it can also damage healthy cells. Chemotherapy can lead to depletion of essential electrolytes and minerals, including sodium, potassium, calcium, and magnesium. Patients should work closely with their healthcare providers because deficiencies in calcium and magnesium can cause symptoms such as muscle cramping and twitching.

It's important to note that taking excessive supplements without medical guidance can lead to serious health issues, including worsening neuropathy (nerve damage). Anyone suspecting a nutrient deficiency should first consult their physician for appropriate testing. After confirming a deficiency, working with a nutrition expert or dietitian can ensure safe and effective supplementation, tailored to individual needs and treatment plans.

Before we dive into recipes, I want to share a little about breast cancer and its treatments. This isn't meant to overwhelm you, it's here to help you feel informed and supported as you move forward.

Breast Cancer Isn't Just One Thing

Breast cancer isn't a single disease. There are different types, based on where it starts and what makes it grow. Knowing these differences helps doctors choose the best treatment for each person.

Most breast cancers aren't linked to inherited genes, but sometimes genetic testing can help guide treatment and show whether family members might be at risk too.

How It's Found

Breast cancer is often discovered when someone notices a change, such as:

- A lump
- Nipple discharge
- An area of skin that looks different (dimpling or redness that doesn't go away)

Other times, it's found during a routine mammogram or breast MRI (especially for women with dense breast tissue or higher risk). To confirm what's going on, doctors usually do a core needle biopsy. This test doesn't just check for cancer. It also tells them:

Tumor grade – how normal or abnormal the cells look

Hormone receptors – whether the cancer grows with estrogen or progesterone

HER2 status – whether the cancer has too much of a protein that makes cells grow

In Situ vs. Invasive Breast Cancer

In Situ

"In situ" means *"in its original place."* These are early changes that haven't spread outside the breast ducts or lobules.

- The most common is ductal carcinoma in situ (DCIS), which can turn into invasive cancer if untreated.
- Another type, lobular carcinoma in situ (LCIS), isn't cancer but signals a higher lifetime risk. Women with LCIS may be advised to take hormone-blocking medication, like tamoxifen, to lower that risk.

Invasive

Invasive cancers have moved beyond the ducts or lobules into the surrounding breast tissue.

- The most common type is invasive ductal carcinoma (IDC), which makes up about 80% of breast cancer cases.
- Invasive cancers can also spread to lymph nodes or other parts of the body if not treated.
- Some invasive cancers grow slowly. These are often hormone receptor-positive (HR+) and HER2-negative.
- They're usually treated with surgery first, followed by years of hormone-blocking medication.
- Doctors now use special tests, like Oncotype, to decide if chemotherapy is really needed.
- Others behave more aggressively.
- They may be hormone receptor-negative (HR-) or HER2-positive.
- These often require treatments like chemotherapy, HER2-targeted drugs, and sometimes immunotherapy before surgery.
- HR+ often carry a better prognosis than HER2-but there are powerful treatments and new breakthroughs bringing hope to everyone.

Targeted Treatments

- **Hormone Therapy** – Medicines like tamoxifen or aromatase inhibitors block hormones, like estrogen, from feeding the cancer.

- **HER2-Targeted Therapy** – Drugs like Herceptin attach to HER2 proteins to stop cancer cells from growing.

Taking Care of Yourself During and After Treatment

Cancer treatment can be tough on your body. While chemotherapy and other drugs fight cancer, they can also lower important minerals like:

- Sodium
- Potassium
- Calcium
- Magnesium

When these drop too low, you might feel muscle cramps, twitching, or extra fatigue. If you notice these symptoms, let your doctor know.

It's tempting to reach for supplements, but more isn't always better. Taking too much of certain vitamins or minerals can cause serious problems, even worsen side effects like nerve pain.

Tip:

Always talk to your doctor before starting supplements.

Supplements may interfere with your treatment. Ask your doctor to check your levels first and work with a nutrition expert to find what's right for you.

Knowledge is power. Understanding the basics can help you feel more in control, and that's an important step toward healing.

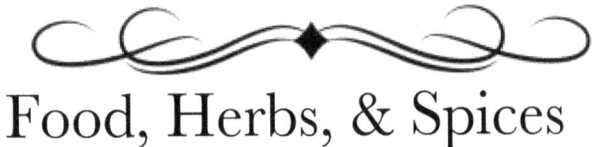

Food, Herbs, & Spices

I spent many days researching food that

inhibits cancer cells from multiplying,

looking at many countries list for foods or

important components that have been

found to reduce the risk of several types

of breast cancer. Throughout the cookbook

I will be sharing the information that I have found.

Incorporate them

into your meals whenever possible.

They are loaded with antioxidants,

flavonoids, and polyphenols and have been

shown through studies to inhibit breast cancer.

Here is a list of the vegetables, fruits,

proteins, beverages, grains, nuts and seeds,

herbs, spices, and oils that have been

found to be helpful in reducing cancer

risk and fighting cell reproduction.

Foods and Spices That May Reduce the Risk of ER+/PR+ Breast Cancer

The following foods, spices, and their important components have been found to potentially reduce the risk of estrogen receptor-positive (ER+) and progesterone receptor-positive (PR+) breast cancer:

Vegetables

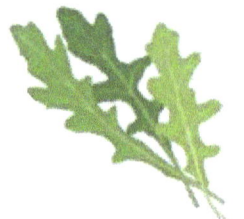

Artichokes

Arugula

Dry Beans

Red Beetroot

Bell Peppers

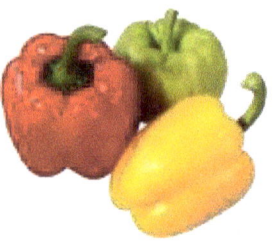

Bok Choy

Broccoli and Broccoli Sprouts

Brussels Sprouts

Butter Beans

Butternut Squash

Cabbage

Carrots

Cauliflower

Celery and Celery Hearts

Collard Greens

Cucumbers

Green Beans (French, Haricot, Runner)

Hot Peppers

Kale

Kidney Beans

Leeks

Romaine Lettuce

Mushrooms (especially White Button, Oyster, Portabella, Lingzhi)

Mustard Greens

Onions (all types)

Pumpkins

Red Chili Peppers

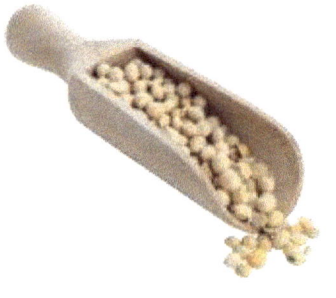

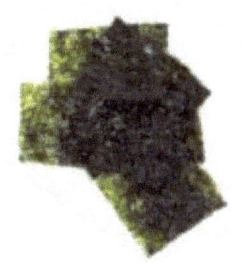

Red Lentils

Seaweed

Tomatoes

Turnips

Watercress and Garden Cress

Zucchini

Nutritional Benefits

These vegetables are rich in vitamins, minerals, fiber, and a variety of phytochemicals that support the body's natural defenses against cancer. Cruciferous vegetables like broccoli, Brussels sprouts, cabbage, and kale contain sulforaphane and indoles, compounds shown to help detoxify carcinogens and regulate estrogen metabolism.

Leafy greens such as collard greens and mustard greens provide high levels of antioxidants like vitamin C and beta-carotene, which reduce oxidative stress and inflammation, key drivers in cancer development. Beans and lentils are excellent sources of plant-based protein and fiber, promoting healthy digestion and hormone regulation. Additionally, vegetables like bell peppers, tomatoes, and carrots offer lycopene and carotenoids, powerful antioxidants linked to lower breast cancer risk.

Fruits

Apples (especially Pink Lady, including apple peel and apple extract)

Pectic Acid (from apples)

Bilberries (Jamun) and Bilberry Extract

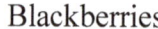

Blackberries

Blueberries

Boysenberries

Cantaloupe

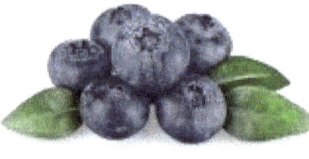

Sweet or Tart Cherries

Cranberries and Cranberry Extract

Black Currants

Red or Purple Grape Juice

Red or Black Grapes (including Vitis amurensis)

Grape Skin Extract (including Muscadine grape skin)

Grapefruit

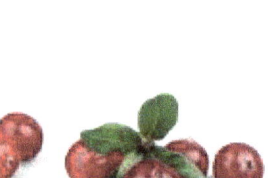

Jujube

Japanese Quince

Lemon

Lingonberries

Lime

Litchi Fruit Pericarp Extract

Mango (including Mango Peel Extract — Nam Doc Mai,
and Mango Seed Ethanolic Extract)

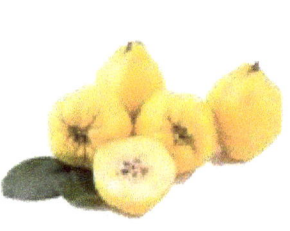

Mangosteen

Orange

Peach

Pineapple Skin and Stem (contains Bromelain)

Immature Plum

Pomelo

Pomegranate Juice, Whole Pomegranates,
Fermented Pomegranate Extract and Seed Oil

Raspberries

Strawberries and Strawberry Methanolic Extract

Watermelon

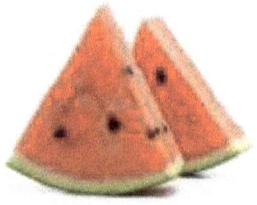

Nutritional Benefits

Fruits on this list are packed with a wide range of cancer-fighting nutrients including polyphenols, flavonoids, and vitamins that help inhibit tumor growth and support immune function. Berries such as blueberries, strawberries, and raspberries are particularly rich in anthocyanins and ellagic acid, which have been shown to reduce inflammation and oxidative damage to DNA.

Apples provide pectin, a type of fiber that supports gut health and may influence estrogen metabolism. Citrus fruits like oranges, lemons, and grapefruit deliver high doses of vitamin C and limonoids, compounds with anti-cancer properties.

Pomegranates are noted for their ellagitannins and punicalagins, potent antioxidants that can inhibit cancer cell proliferation and induce apoptosis (programmed cell death). Tropical fruits like mango and pineapple add digestive enzymes such as bromelain, which support immune response and reduce inflammation.

Overall, these fruits contribute to hormonal balance and create a biological environment less favorable for ER+/PR+ breast cancer development.

Protein Sources

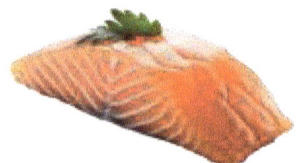

Arctic Char

Chicken (organic)

Turkey (organic)

Salmon (wild)

Herring

Lake Trout

Mackerel

Sardines

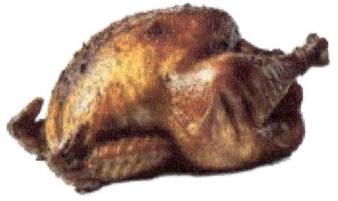

Nutritional Benefits

Wild-caught fish such as salmon, mackerel, trout, and sardines are excellent sources of omega-3 fatty acids, which help reduce inflammation, support hormone balance, and may inhibit the growth of hormone-sensitive tumors. They also provide vitamin D and selenium, which support immune and cellular health. Organic poultry (chicken and turkey) offers clean, lean protein without the added hormones or antibiotics found in conventionally raised meat, supporting overall health during cancer prevention or treatment.

Whole Grains, Beverages, Nuts & Seeds

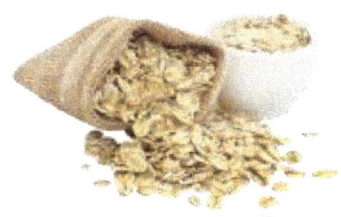

Barley

Buckwheat

Flaxseed

Flaxseed Oil

Oats (whole)

Rice (brown, black, or wild)

Sorghum

Walnuts

Walnut Oil

Wheat (organic)

Carrot Juice (Balero or Betasweet varieties)

Kefir

Green Tea

Nutritional Benefits

Whole grains like oats, barley, brown rice, and sorghum are rich in fiber, which helps regulate estrogen levels by aiding in hormone excretion through digestion. Grains also contain lignans and plant sterols, which may have anti-estrogenic effects. Flaxseeds are particularly powerful, offering lignans and ALA (alpha-linolenic acid), a plant-based omega-3. Walnuts provide polyphenols and healthy fats that support brain, heart, and cellular health.

Carrot juice is high in beta-carotene, a precursor to vitamin A that acts as an antioxidant. Kefir, a probiotic-rich fermented dairy drink, supports gut health, which is increasingly recognized as a factor in estrogen metabolism and immune regulation. Green tea contains EGCG (epigallocatechin gallate), a potent antioxidant shown in lab studies to reduce tumor growth and block angiogenesis.

Herbs, Spices & Oils

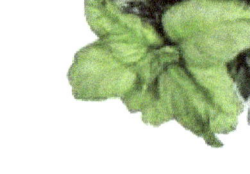

Basil

Black Cumin

Black Cumin Oil

Black Pepper (Piperine)

Cilantro

Fresh Garlic

Ginger

Horseradish

Wasabi

Mustard

Olive Oil (extra virgin)

Olives Oregano

Parsley

Saffron

Thyme

Turmeric

Nutritional Benefits

Many herbs and spices in this list, such as turmeric, black cumin, garlic, and ginger, have well-documented anti-inflammatory and antioxidant properties. Turmeric, in particular, contains curcumin, which may inhibit estrogen receptor activity and reduce tumor growth. Black cumin (and its oil) contains thymoquinone, a compound that has shown anti-cancer potential in several studies.

Olive oil (extra virgin) and olives provide monounsaturated fats and polyphenols that reduce inflammation and oxidative stress. Garlic, wasabi, horseradish, and mustard are high in isothiocyanates and organosulfur compounds, which promote detoxification and may induce cancer cell death. Herbs like oregano, parsley, cilantro, and basil are rich in flavonoids and other plant compounds that support cellular repair and modulate immune responses.

CANCER AND MINDFULNESS

The Power of Mindset

Facing cancer is not only a physical journey, it's an emotional and mental one. And in that journey, your mindset can become one of your most powerful tools. Mindfulness, the practice of staying present and grounded in the moment, helps you respond to the realities of illness with clarity, calm, and inner strength.

One powerful shift begins with language. Instead of saying, "I have cancer," try reframing it as, "I have been diagnosed with cancer." It may seem small, but this change reinforces a vital truth: cancer is an experience you are going through; it is not your identity. You are still whole, worthy, and powerful, regardless of what this diagnosis may suggest.

Your thoughts carry weight.

A positive, resilient mindset doesn't require ignoring fear, sadness, or frustration. These emotions are real and valid. But mindfulness teaches us that we can acknowledge difficulty without letting it define our reality. There will be hard days. There may be pain, grief, or uncertainty. But none of that is permanent. You are allowed to feel it all and still choose hope.

Celebrate even the smallest victories. Whether it's getting out of bed, making it to an appointment, or simply breathing through a difficult moment, every act of courage matters. Focus on what you can control: your breath, your nutrition, your rest, your words, your support system. Surround yourself with people who uplift and encourage you. Let their love remind you of your resilience.

Mindfulness also extends to how you care for your body. Nourishing yourself with healing foods, moving gently when possible, and resting when needed are all sacred acts of self-respect. Each bite of nutrient-rich food is a quiet declaration: "I am choosing to support my healing."Each glass of water, each moment of stillness, each deep breath is a step toward wellness.

Remember:you are not just surviving, you are overcoming. You are adapting, healing, and growing stronger in ways you may not yet see. Let mindfulness anchor you. Let it help you notice the beauty in small things, the strength in your own heart, and the presence of grace in the midst of hardship.

Believe in your ability to heal. Believe that you can find peace, even in uncertainty.

You are not alone.

You are deeply capable.

You've got this.

To ensure people with cancer get the nutrients their bodies need to recover, Kimmel Cancer Center Gabrielle Judd recommends smoothies to boost calorie, protein, and micronutrient intake. Additionally, chemotherapy and radiation may have side effects that make eating difficult, including nausea and dry mouth. Getting fluids and nutrients is important for healing. Looking to boost your calcium as advised by your physician? Try blending plain, unsweetened yogurt into your smoothie.

Remember, you can use fresh or frozen fruits and vegetables, but don't forget to wash any fresh fruits or vegetables well by rubbing them under cold running water before adding them to the blender!

This helps get rid of the bacteria that may be on these foods and promotes overall food safety, which is very important, especially when your immune system is low during cancer treatment. You can also use a vegetable scrubber to help clean anything with thick skin

Change your mind to change your health!

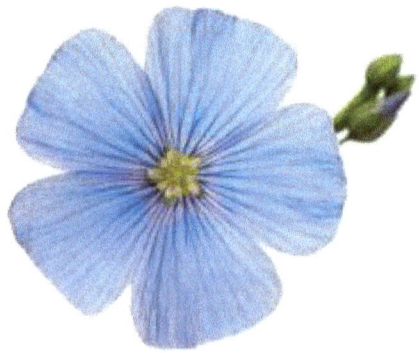

Smoothies

I really love these smoothies! They are full of flavor and are easily made in minutes.

Your body will love you for this.

HOW TO SHAKE IT UP YOUR OWN

Step 1: Begin with Core Shake Ingredients

- 1-2 Scoops High-Quality Protein Powder.

Your powder should be between 15-25g of protein, less than 6g of carbohydrate, less than 2 g of sugar, and preferably at least 2 g of dietary fiber. I like pea protein. Please choose a great protein powder!

- 1 Tablespoon of Flaxseed.

This adds some healthy omega-3s and fiber to your shake.

- 1/3 Cup (or less) of recommended Fruit (Optional).

- See the above list for the best choices.

- 4-8+ Ounces Dairy-Free Liquid.

You may use one liquid alone or a combination of two different liquids (i.e., half water and half unsweetened almond milk). Less liquid may be used if you prefer a thicker consistency shake. Add more liquid if you prefer a thinner consistency shake. Dairy-free liquid choices include:

- Water

- Unsweetened Plain Coconut Milk

- Unsweetened Plain Almond Milk

- Canned Full-Fat Coconut Milk

- Chilled Herbal Tea

Step 2: Choose Any of the Following Smoothie Add-In Options

The add-ins will provide additional nourishment to your smoothie. Adding nutrients in the form of fiber and/or fat will help keep you satiated for several hours! I recommend you choose at least two items from the list below:

● ½-1 Ripe Avocado (makes it so smooth)

● 1 Tbs Flaxseed Oil or Black Cumin Oil

● Additional Chia Seeds (soaked or un-soaked)

● 1 Tbs Barlean's Flavored Omega Swirl (http://www.barleans.com/omega-swirl.asp)

● 1 Tbsp Hemp Seeds

● 1 Tbsp Unsweetened Coconut Flakes

● 1 Tbs Melted Coconut Oil

● Lemon or Lime rind or juice

● 1-2 Raw Pasture Eggs, extra flavoring

● ½-1-ounce walnuts or walnut oil

● 1 Tbsp Cinnamon or 1 Tbsp nut or seed butter

● 1 scoop of Greens or Reds

Step 3: Blend and Enjoy!

You may also consider adding:

● Additional Water or Ice, depending on how thick or thin you like your shake

● 1 Tbs organic Cocoa or Cacao Powder or cocoa nibs for an added chocolate flavoring

● Stevia to taste

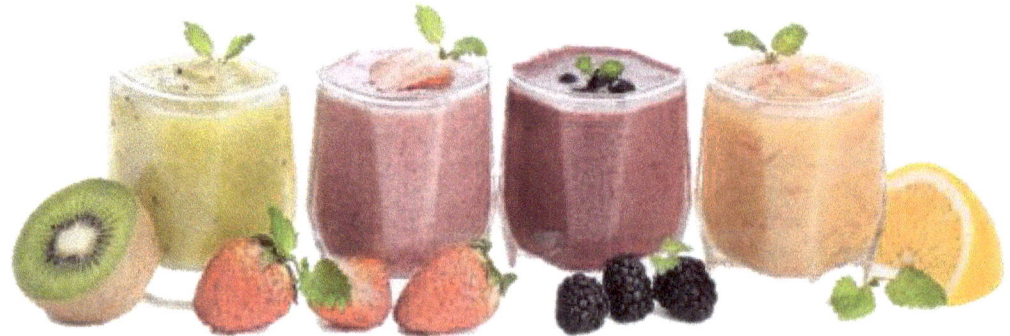

Stevia

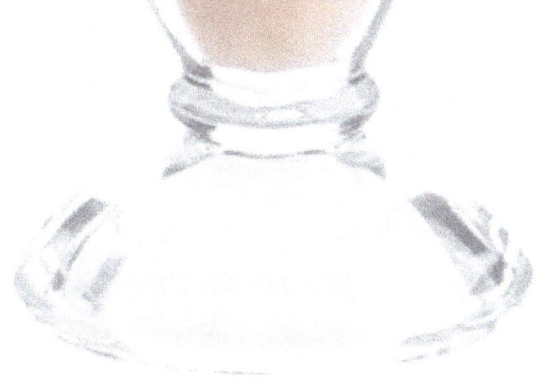

Evidence from emerging research suggests that stevia, a natural sweetener derived from the *Stevia rebaudiana* plant, may offer potential anti-cancer properties, particularly due to its active compounds known as steviol glycosides. These glycosides, including stevioside and rebaudioside A, have demonstrated cytotoxic effects against certain cancer cell lines in laboratory studies.

Preclinical studies have found that steviol glycosides may help inhibit the proliferation of breast cancer cells, induce apoptosis (programmed cell death), and potentially interfere with pathways that support tumor growth. In some cases, these compounds were observed to slow or block the growth of estrogen-receptor-positive (ER+) breast cancer cells, making stevia of interest in hormone-sensitive cancers.

Beyond breast cancer, lab-based research also suggests that stevia's glycosides may exhibit toxic effects against other types of cancer cells, including those from the stomach (gastric), lung, and certain leukemias. These effects are believed to occur through mechanisms like oxidative stress induction, DNA fragmentation, and disruption of mitochondrial function, which impair the cancer cells' ability to survive and multiply.

However, it's important to note that most of this research has been conducted in vitro (in test tubes) or in animal models, and human clinical studies are still limited. While promising, stevia should not be viewed as a standalone treatment for cancer, but rather as a potentially supportive dietary component within a broader, evidence-based approach to health and nutrition.

Replacing sugar with natural, non-caloric sweeteners like stevia can also help manage blood glucose levels, reduce insulin resistance, and lower chronic inflammation, all of which are factors that may contribute to a lower cancer risk over time.

The Power of Mangoes

A fascinating study compared three genetically diverse mango varieties, like Irwin, Kensington Pride, and Nam Doc Mai, to evaluate their effects on human breast cancer cells. The researchers found that the peel extract from the Nam Doc Mai mango contained the highest levels of polyphenols, particularly soluble compounds known for their antioxidant and anticancer properties ([era.dpi.qld.gov.au](era.dpi.qld.gov.au)).

When tested on two breast cancer cell lines, like MCF-7 (ER-positive) and MDA-MB-231 (triple-negative), theNam Doc Mai peel extract significantly inhibited cell viability, with an IC_{50} of around 56 µg/mL for MCF-7, and triggered cancer cell death ($p < 0.01$) in MDA-MB-231 cells ([era.dpi.qld.gov.au](era.dpi.qld.gov.au)).

These robust effects were linked to the high polyphenol content unique to Nam Doc Mai peel, such as gallic acid, galloylated derivatives, and methyl gallate, compounds effective at inducing apoptosis and suppressing proliferation in aggressive breast cancer cells (pmc.ncbi.nlm.nih.gov). While much of the research is still at the lab stage, these promising findings highlight mango peel, especially from the Nam Doc Mai variety, as a rich source of plant nutrients that may offer protective and therapeutic benefits against breast cancer.

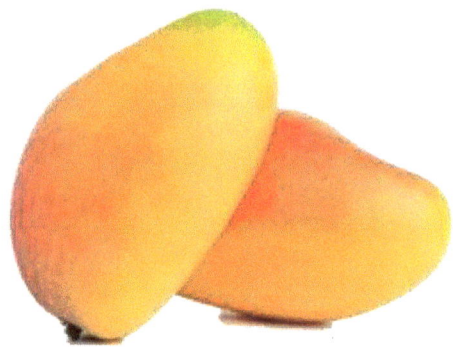

Mango Shake

YIELD: 1 SERVING

Love the burst of fresh flavor from mangos with just a bit of coconut? This shake is full of flavor, and packed with protein, fiber, and healthy fats.

Ingredients

1 serving Protein Powder (Choose a protein powder that prioritizes purity- free of preservatives, dyes and artificial flavors.)

½ c. Unsweetened, Plain Almond Milk

1/4 c. Walnuts

½ c. Canned Full-Fat Coconut Milk 4 Ice Cubes

½ Kiwi, peeled

2 Tbsp. Flax Seeds

2 tsp. Stevia (optional)

Instructions

Place all ingredients in the blender.

Add approximately ½ cup of water to create the desired consistency.

Process until smooth.

Serve Immediately.

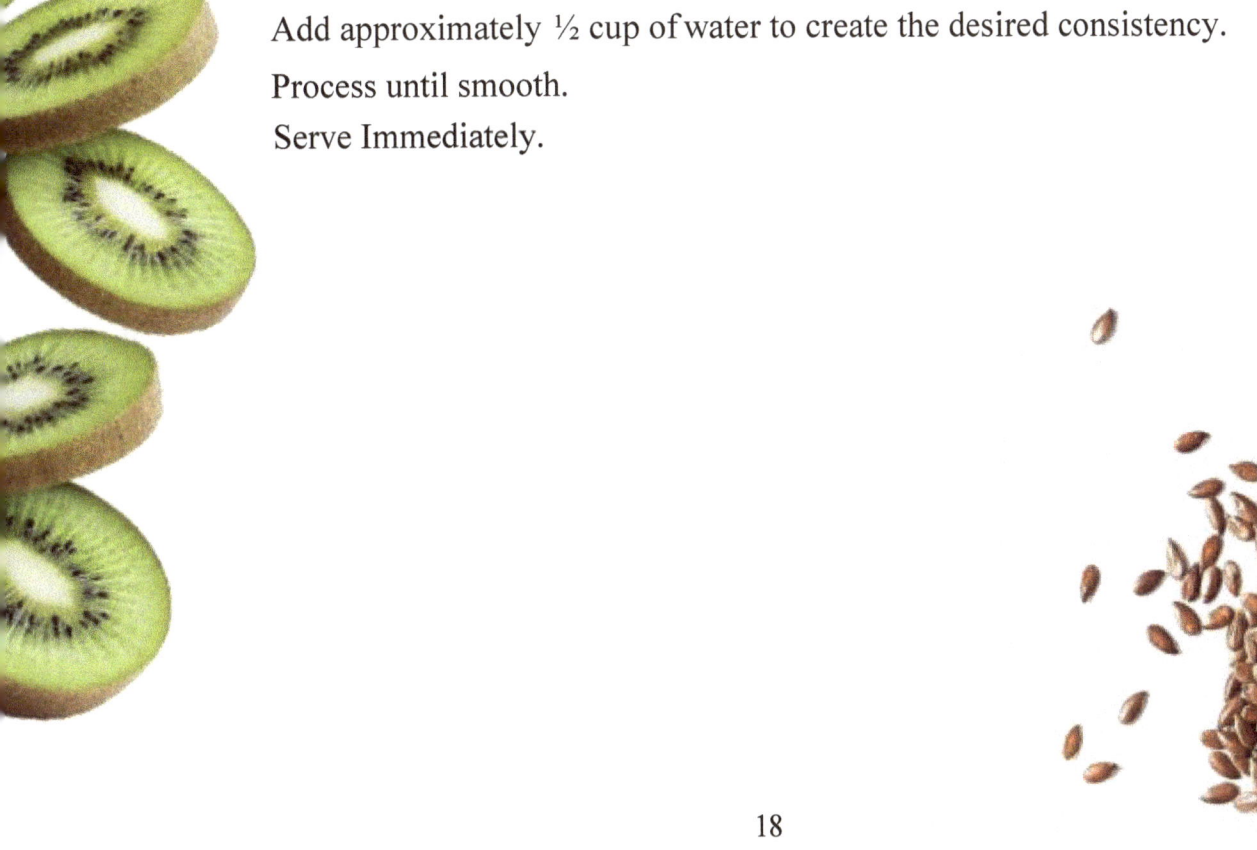

Apple Strudel Shake

YIELD: 1 SERVING

Cinnamon, apples, and walnuts make this fragrant breakfast shake taste just like a freshly baked strudel. For spice lovers, add a pinch of ground clove or pumpkin spice for extra warmth.

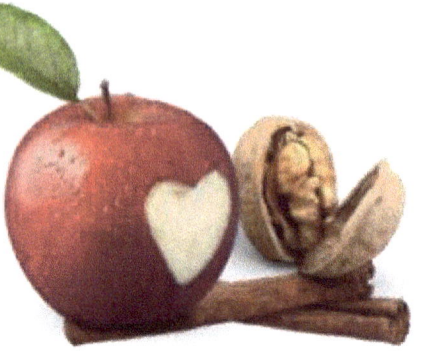

Ingredients

1 serving protein powder
½ tsp. ground cinnamon
⅓ cup chopped apple (peel on)
1 Tbsp. flaxseed
½ cup unsweetened plain almond milk *or* water
2 Tbsp. chopped walnuts
½ cup canned full-fat coconut milk
½ tsp. vanilla bean paste
4 ice cubes
Pinch of ground clove *or* pumpkin spice (optional)
2 tsp. powdered stevia *or* 5—12 drops liquid stevia (optional)
½ avocado (optional, for creaminess)

Instructions

Place all ingredients in a blender.

Add about ½ cup of water to adjust to your desired consistency.

Blend until smooth.
Serve immediately.

Nutrition Note

Apples are one of the most widely consumed fruits worldwide and have long been celebrated for their nutritional value and health-promoting properties. Rich in fiber, vitamins, minerals, and bioactive compounds, apples play a beneficial role in maintaining overall wellness and may offer protection against chronic diseases, including certain types of cancer. Recent scientific research has highlighted apples as a functional food with potential anti-cancer properties, particularly due to their high content of phytochemicals, naturally occurring plant compounds with biological activity.

Flavonoids and Breast Cancer

One of the key classes of bioactive compounds found in apples is flavonoids, which are potent antioxidants and anti-inflammatory agents. These compounds are especially concentrated in the skin of the apple, making it important to consume apples with the peel on.

Studies focusing on Pink Lady apples, for instance, have shown that flavonoid extracts from both the peel and flesh can inhibit the proliferation of MCF-7 breast cancer cells in vitro. This inhibition is thought to be linked to the ability of flavonoids to interfere with cancer cell signaling pathways, reduce oxidative DNA damage, and regulate enzymes involved in cell cycle control.

Pectic Acid and Metastasis Prevention

Apples are also a significant source of **pectin**, a type of soluble fiber, and its derivative, pectic acid, has demonstrated notable anti-cancer effects. In laboratory studies, pectic acid has been shown to:

- Induce apoptosis (programmed cell death) in cancer cells
- Inhibit the growth of 4T1 breast cancer cells (a model for triple-negative breast cancer)
- Prevent tumor metastasis, which is the spread of cancer from its original site to other parts of the body.

These effects are believed to result from pectic acid's ability to bind to and block galectin-3, a protein involved in tumor progression and metastasis. By disrupting this pathway, pectic substances from apples may slow the spread of cancer and support the body's natural immune defenses.

Other Health-Promoting Compounds in Apples

In addition to flavonoids and pectic acid, apples contain a variety of other nutrients and plant compounds that contribute to their health benefits:

- **Quercetin**: A well-known flavonoid that can reduce inflammation, fight free radicals, and modulate immune function
- **Catechins**: Antioxidants also found in green tea that support heart and brain health and may help inhibit tumor formation
- **Chlorogenic acid**: A polyphenol that may help regulate blood sugar and protect DNA from oxidative damage
- **Dietary fiber**: Supports gut health, regulates blood sugar levels, and plays a role in detoxification.

While apples alone are not a cure or guarantee against cancer, their regular inclusion in a balanced, plant-rich diet may contribute to reduced cancer risk and improved long-term health. Consuming whole apples with the peel intact maximizes the intake of beneficial compounds. Choosing a variety of apple types may also provide a broader spectrum of phytonutrients.

Emerging research continues to reinforce the wisdom of the old saying: *"An apple a day keeps the doctor away."* In the context of cancer prevention and overall health, that advice
may be more relevant than ever.

Chocolate Walnut Crunch Shake

Sweet blueberries and rich dark chocolate make this shake both delicious and antioxidant-rich. You can use fresh or frozen berries; frozen tends to be more budget-friendly.

Ingredients

1 serving protein powder
½ cup canned coconut milk
1 Tbsp unsweetened dark organic cocoa powder
4 ice cubes
⅓ cup blueberries
1 Tbsp ground flaxseed
1 Tbsp walnuts
1–2 tsp stevia powder or 5–12 drops liquid (optional)
½ avocado (optional)

Instructions

Place all ingredients in a blender.
Add approximately ½ cup of water
to reach your preferred consistency.

Blend until smooth.
Serve immediately

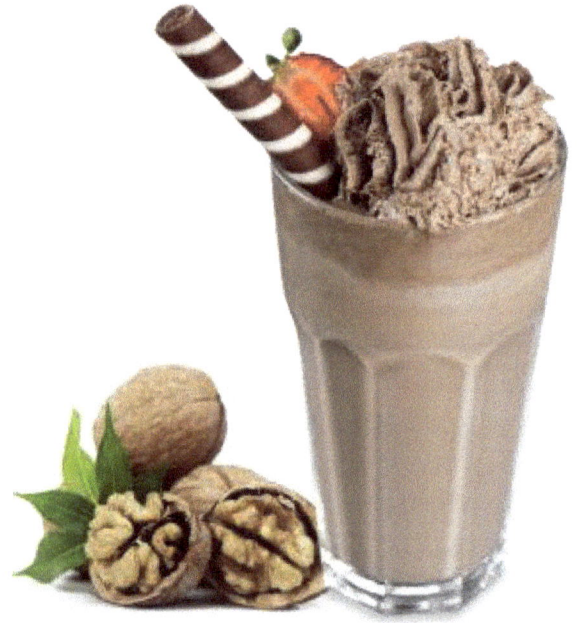

Nutrition Note

Cancer has long been viewed primarily as a disease driven by genetic mutations, either inherited or acquired. However, growing evidence suggests that cancer is not solely a genetic inevitability. Instead, many cases may be largely preventable through lifestyle and dietary choices. It is now well established that chronic inflammation, oxidative stress, and hormonal imbalances all play significant roles in the development and progression of cancer.

Dietary factors, in particular, have been shown to influence cancer risk profoundly. Among various foods studied for their protective properties, walnuts have emerged as a promising functional food with potential anti-cancer effects.

Walnuts contain a unique combination of nutrients and phytochemicals, including:

- **Omega-3 fatty acids**: Anti-inflammatory fats that may help reduce the risk of certain cancers by suppressing tumor growth and promoting healthy cell function.

- **Tocopherols (Vitamin E compounds)**: Powerful antioxidants that protect cells from oxidative damage, a known contributor to cancer development.

- **β-Sitosterol**: A plant sterol that inhibits cancer cell growth and promotes apoptosis (programmed cell death), particularly in hormone-related cancers such as breast and prostate cancer.

- **Pedunculagin**: A polyphenol with antioxidant and anti-inflammatory properties that may inhibit angiogenesis (the formation of new blood vessels that feed tumors) and prevent metastasis (the spread of cancer).

In addition to these compounds, walnuts are rich in polyphenols and fiber, both of which support gut health, modulate the immune system, and may contribute to lower cancer risk.

Emerging research from both animal studies and clinical trials continues to support the role of walnuts in cancer prevention. For example, some studies have shown that diets enriched with walnuts can slow the growth of breast and prostate tumors in animal models while improving biomarkers of inflammation and oxidative stress in humans. While no single food can prevent cancer on its own, incorporating nutrient-dense foods like walnuts into a balanced, plant-forward diet may play a meaningful role in reducing overall cancer risk

Cherry Amaretto Shake

YIELD: 1 SERVING

Walnuts and cherries in this recipe taste like cherry pie. Kale might seem like a strange addition, but you won't taste it, and you'll reap its nutritional benefits like fiber, folate, vitamin C, and more.

Ingredients

1 serving protein powder
½ cup unsweetened plain almond milk
½ cup canned full-fat coconut milk
4 ice cubes
¼ cup cherries (fresh or frozen)
1 Tbsp ground flaxseed
¼ cup baby kale leaves (optional)
2 tsp stevia powder or 5—12 drops liquid
¼ tsp almond extract (optional)
2 Tbsp chopped walnuts

Instructions

Place all ingredients in a blender.
Add approximately ½ cup of water to achieve the desired consistency.

Blend until smooth.
Serve immediately.

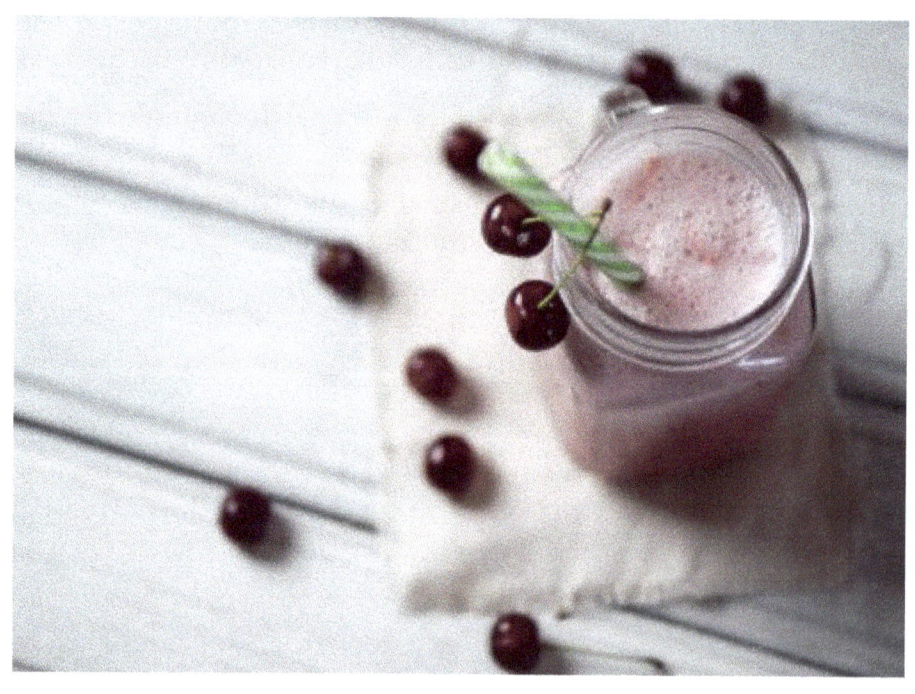

Black Forest Cherry Cake Shake

YIELD: 1 SERVING

Black Forest cake is known for its decadent blend of dark chocolate and cherries. This shake captures the same flavors with nutrient-rich ingredients. Sweet dark cherries combine with cocoa nibs (100% crushed cocoa bean) for a rich chocolate kick. If cocoa nibs aren't available, you can substitute unsweetened cocoa powder mixed with a touch of coconut oil.

Ingredients:

1 serving protein powder

⅓ cup frozen cherries

¼ cup baby spinach

½ cup unsweetened almond milk or coconut milk

4 ice cubes (crushed)

2 Tbsp flaxseeds

1 Tbsp cocoa nibs (or unsweetened cocoa powder + ½ tsp coconut oil)

½ tsp almond or vanilla extract

Instructions:

Place all ingredients in a blender.

Blend until smooth and creamy.

Serve immediately and enjoy.

Coconut Chai Shake

Chai tea is loved worldwide for its warm, comforting flavors. The blend of cinnamon, nutmeg, and cardamom not only enhances taste but also provides valuable minerals like manganese and calcium. Combined with coconut, this shake is both nourishing and delicious.

Ingredients:

1 serving protein powder
1 carrot, chopped
½ cup unsweetened coconut milk (from carton, not canned)
¼ cup shredded unsweetened organic coconut
4 ice cubes (crushed)
2 Tbsp flaxseeds
½ tsp vanilla extract
½ tsp cinnamon
¼ tsp cardamom and/or nutmeg

Instructions:

Place all ingredients in a blender.
Add ½ cup water.
Blend until smooth and creamy.
Serve immediately and enjoy.

Stay hydrated, opt for fruits, whole grains ,and lean protein, and try to eat snacks and smaller meals throughout your day instead of larger portions.

Salted Dark Chocolate Shake

YIELD: 1 SERVING

Sweet and salty make an irresistible combination, and this shake delivers just that. Chia and flaxseeds add thickness and crunch, while dark chocolate brings a powerful dose ofantioxidants and superfood nutrients.

Ingredients:
1 serving protein powder
½ cup kale, chopped
½ cup unsweetened almond or coconut milk (from carton, not canned)
4 ice cubes (crushed)
1 Tbsp cocoa powder
2 Tbsp flaxseeds
½ tsp vanilla bean paste
½ tsp cinnamon
⅛ tsp sea salt
2 Tbsp cocoa nibs
½ avocado
1 tsp stevia or 5–15 drops
chocolate or coconut stevia (optional)

Instructions:
Place all ingredients in a blender, except cocoa nibs.
Blend until smooth and creamy.

Stir in the cocoa nibs for texture.
Serve immediately.

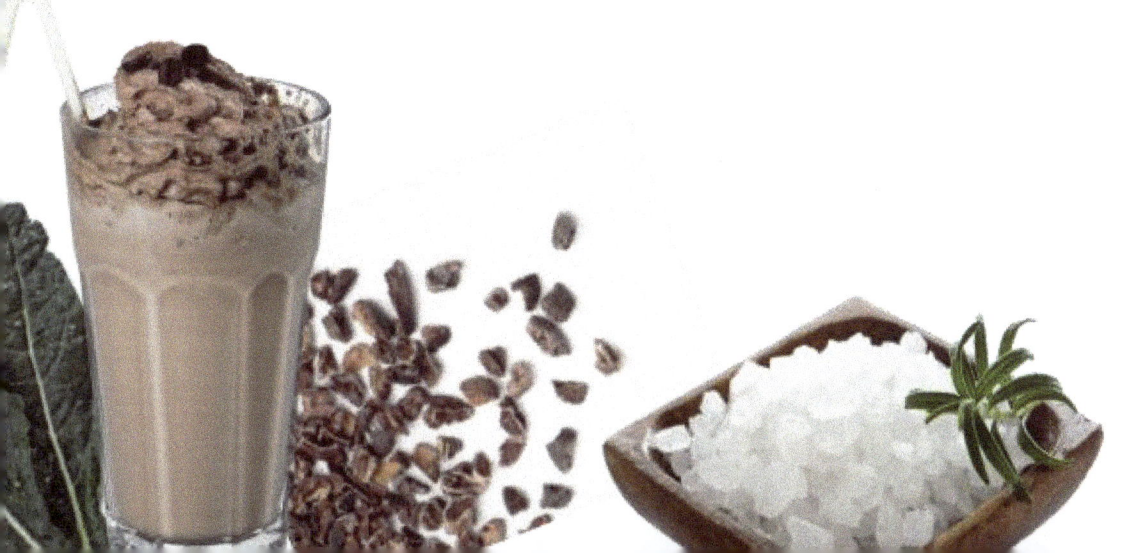

Choco-Almo Shake

YIELD: 1 SERVING

This rich chocolate shake, combined with almond butter, tastes like a candy bar!

Ingredients:

1 serving protein powder

1 cup unsweetened almond milk or coconut milk

1 Tbsp almond butter

1 heaping Tbsp raw cocoa or cocoa nibs

1 Tbsp flaxseed

½ avocado

5–15 drops of chocolate stevia (adjust to taste)

Instructions:

Add all ingredients to a blender.

Blend until smooth.

Serve immediately.

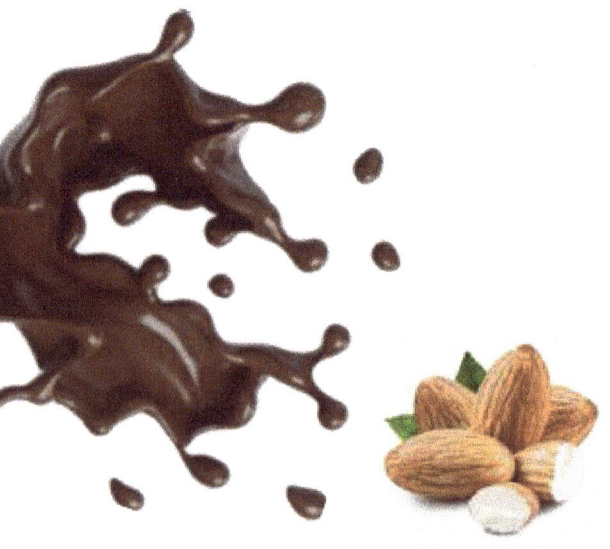

Health Spotlight

Flaxseed is a tiny nutritional powerhouse that offers a wide range of health benefits, particularly for hormone-related cancers like breast and prostate cancer.

Cancer Prevention & Hormonal Health:

Several studies have shown that consuming 25 grams (about 2 tablespoons) of ground flaxseed daily may significantly reduce tumor growth, especially in hormone-sensitive cancers such as breast and prostate cancer. This effect is primarily due to flaxseed's high content of lignans, plant compounds that have antioxidant and phytoestrogenic properties, meaning they can help balance hormone levels in the body.

In the case of breast cancer, flaxseed consumption has been linked to:

A reduction in estrogen production which may lower the risk of estrogen receptor-positive (ER+) breast cancers.

Slowed tumor growth in early-stage breast cancer.

Enhanced the effectiveness of tamoxifen, a drug widely used in hormone therapy to prevent breast cancer recurrence. Research suggests that flaxseed may increase the anti-tumor action of tamoxifen, making it a valuable complementary dietary addition during treatment (with medical supervision).

For prostate cancer, studies have shown:

Reduced tumor proliferation.

Improved markers of cancer progression when flaxseed is included as part of a low-fat, plant-based diet.

Other Health Benefits of Flaxseed Include:

- Rich in Omega-3s: Flaxseed is one of the best plant-based sources of alpha-linolenic acid (ALA), an essential omega-3 fatty acid known for its anti-inflammatory properties.
- High in Fiber: Supports digestive health, helps maintain regularity, and may aid in weight management by promoting satiety.
- Heart Health: May reduce blood pressure, improve cholesterol levels, and lower the risk of cardiovascular disease.
- Blood Sugar Control: The soluble fiber in flaxseed helps regulate blood sugar levels, making it beneficial for people with diabetes or insulin resistance.

Tip for Best Results:

Flaxseed is best consumed ground rather than whole, as whole seeds may pass through the digestive system undigested. Store ground flaxseed in the refrigerator or freezer in an airtight container to prevent oxidation and preserve its nutrient content.

CARROT CAKE SHAKE

1 SERVING

Ingredients

- 1 serving protein powder
- 1 carrot, chopped
- ¼ cup apple (skin on), chopped
- ½ cup unsweetened almond milk or coconut milk
- 4 ice cubes (crushed)
- 1 Tbsp chopped walnuts
- 1 Tbsp flaxseeds
- 1 Tbsp orange zest
- ½ tsp vanilla extract
- ½ tsp cinnamon
- ½ tsp nutmeg

Instructions

1. Place all ingredients in a blender.
2. Blend until smooth.
3. Serve immediately

Raspberry Lime Shake

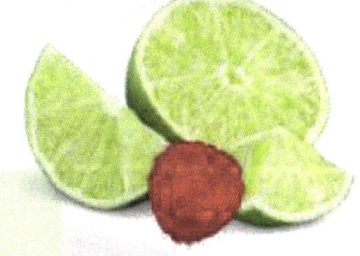

YIELD: 1 SERVING

Try kefir with this recipe. It's incredibly beneficial for gut health and adds a tangy, creamy twist. Raspberries provide vitamin C and fiber, while spinach brings a wealth of nutrients like vitamins A, C, K1, folic acid, iron, calcium, and insoluble fiber.

Ingredients

1 serving protein powder

8 oz kefir

½ cup frozen raspberries

Juice and zest of ½ lime

1 Tbsp flaxseeds

1 large handful baby spinach

12–25 drops lime stevia (optional)

4 ice cubes (crushed)

½ cup water

Instructions:

Place all ingredients in a blender.

Blend until smooth.
Serve immediately.

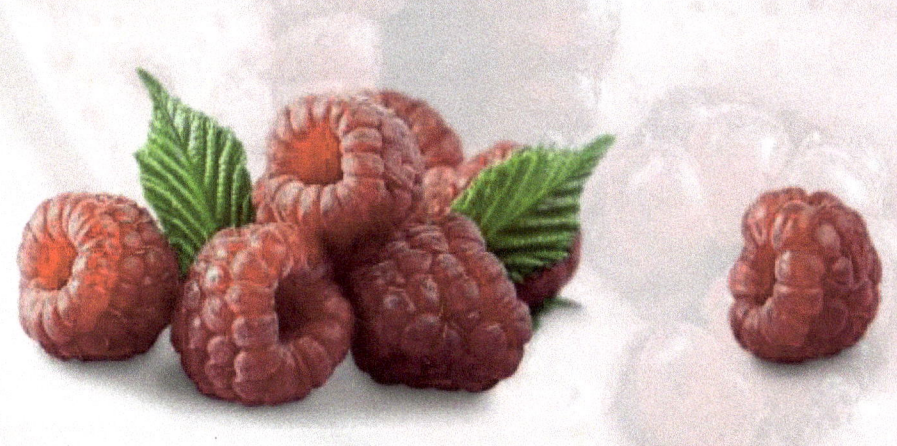

Orange Crush

A refreshing fusion of fruits, protein, and warm spices.
Cinnamon and nutmeg add antioxidant power, while the burst of citrus provides vitamin C to energize your body and support immunity.

Ingredients

1 serving Vanilla Protein Powder (soy-free)
1 medium carrot, peeled and chopped
¼ cup apple, chopped (skin-on for fiber)
1 small orange, peeled and seeded
½ cup brewed Constant Comment tea (cooled) *or*
unsweetened coconut milk
4 ice cubes, crushed
1 Tbsp. walnuts, chopped
1 Tbsp. ground flax seeds
1 Tbsp. orange zest
½ tsp. vanilla paste *or* vanilla extract
½ tsp. ground cinnamon
¼ tsp. ground nutmeg
Optional: 1 tsp. honey or stevia for extra sweetness

Instructions

Place all ingredients in a blender.
Blend until smooth, adding a splash of water or extra coconut milk if needed for the desired consistency.
Serve immediately, chilled.

Vitamin C from oranges can also boost the absorption of iron from foods.

This helps protect against anemia, a common side effect of cancer therapies.

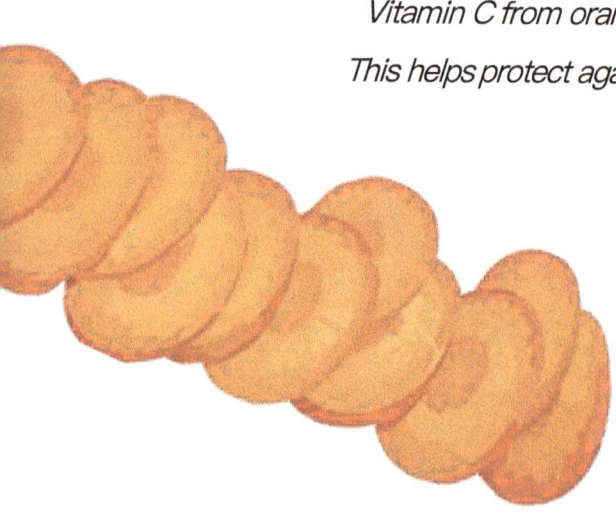

31

Peachy Nutmeg Shake

YIELD: 1 SERVING

These Are A Few Of My Favorite Things. Just Wow!

A creamy, peachy shake that's simple, refreshing, and packed with nourishing ingredients.
Perfect as a post-workout refuel or a guilt-free treat.

Ingredients

1 Serving Protein Powder No Soy

8 Oz. Unsweetened Almond Or Coconut Milk
½ C. Frozen Peaches
½ Tsp. Nutmeg
1 Tbsp. Flax Seeds
Peach Stevia Drops 5-20

Instructions

Add all ingredients to the blender
Blend until very smooth.

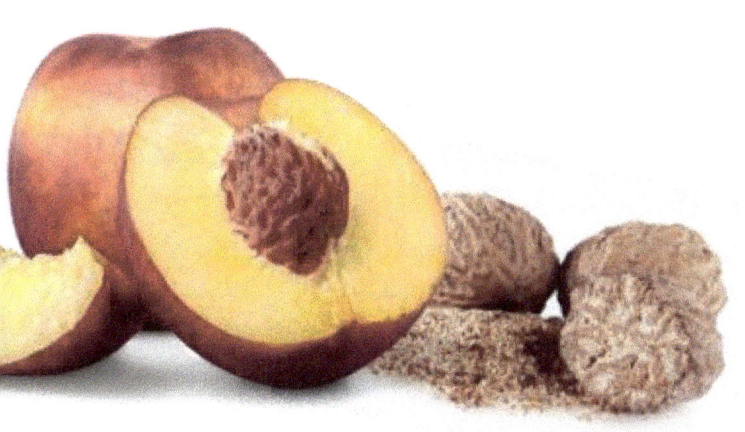

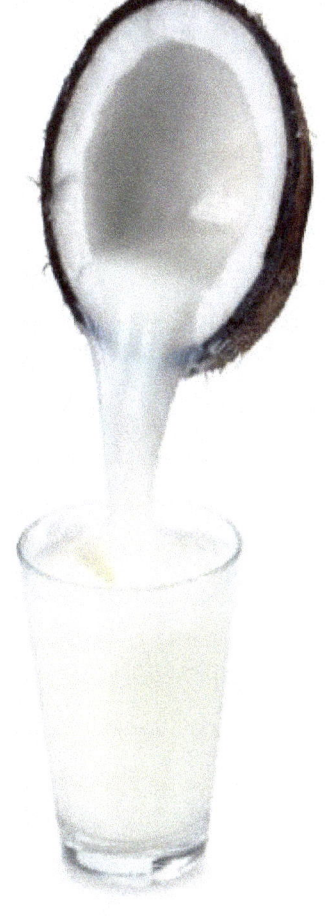

MOCHA FUDGE SHAKE

YIELD: 1 SERVING

So stinking good, you will think that you are cheating!
Just the right combination to satisfy that chocolate and coffee craving.

Ingredients

½ C. coconut milk
½ C. rich coffee
1 Tbsp. cocoa nibs
1 Tbsp. organic cocoa
1 Tbsp. walnuts
1 Tbsp. chia seeds
1 Tbsp.
4 ice cubes (Crushed)

Instructions

Add all ingredients in the order listed.
Blend until very well mixed.
Add crushed ice and blend until smooth.

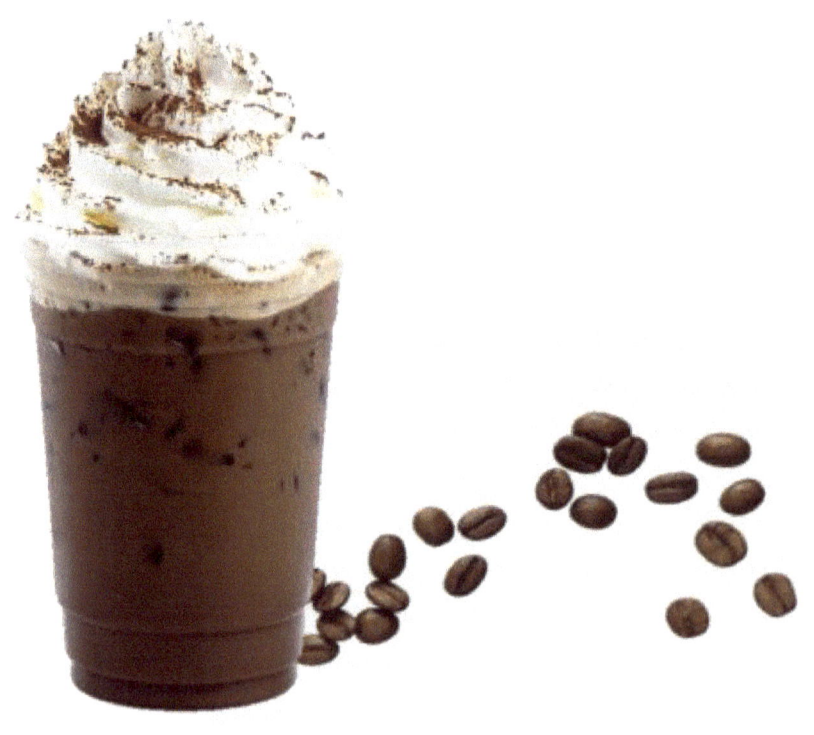

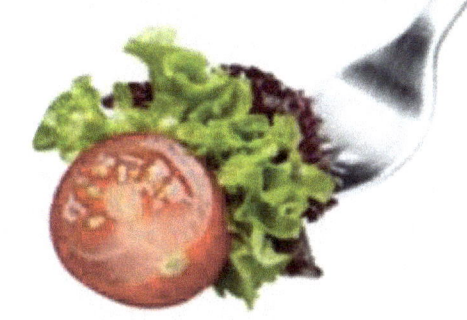

Salad

Cruciferous Vegetables

Have Shown To Inhibit The Growth Of Breast Cancer Cells

Benzyl isothiocyanate (BITC) induced

inhibition of breast cancer cells. Benzyl

isothiocyanate (BITC) is a naturally occurring

compoundfound inplants like mustard, broccoli,

cabbage, and watercress, belonging

to the mustardfamily, and is known for its

potential anticancerproperties due to

its ability to induce cell death (apoptosis) in

cancer cells; it is currently being studied for its

potential as a chemopreventive agent against

various cancers.

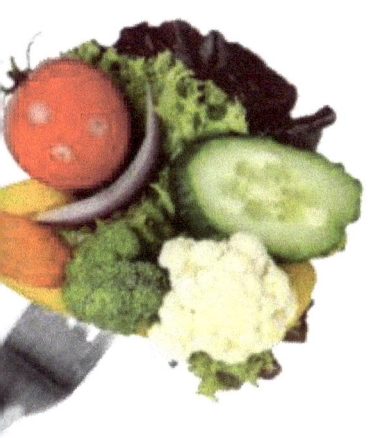

Create You Own Salad

Set up a salad bar at home using the following ingredients,
or substitute with your own favorites.
Prep portioned storage containers in your fridge,
so your salad bar is ready any time you open your fridge.

Suggested Base

Tomatoes

4 c. Romaine Lettuce, Arugula,Kale- chopped

1 c. Green Beans, steamed

1 c. Broccoli Florets, raw

Cauliflower

Celery

Cabbage

Carrots

Mushrooms

Onions

1 c. Artichokes, quartered

Cucumbers

Suggested Toppings

Protein of your choice (chicken, turkey, eggs, fish)

½ c. Pitted Black or Green Olives

1 Avocado

½ oz. nuts (i.e., walnuts, flax seeds)

1 c. bean sprouts

Butternut Squash

Carrots

Instructions

Mix and match from the base and toppings
category to make the salad of your choice!

Serve with one of the recommended dressings

Salad Dressings

Lime Dressing
1 Lime, zested and juiced (about 2 Tbsp.)
1 Tbsp.EVOO oil
1 tsp. Dijon mustard
A few drops of liquid stevia (to taste)

Instructions:
Whisk all ingredients together until smooth.

Lemon Vinaigrette
A light, refreshing classic that pairs with almost any salad.
¼ cup fresh lemon juice
¼ cup extra-virgin olive oil
¼ tsp. sea salt
¼ tsp. freshly ground black pepper

Instructions
Combine ingredients in a small bowl or jar. Whisk or shake until emulsified.

Greek Dressing
A savory, Mediterranean-style dressing full of bold flavors.

¼ cup walnut oil *or* extra-virgin olive oil
3 Tbsp. fresh lemon juice
1 clove garlic, finely minced
½ tsp. dried oregano
¼ tsp. Dijon mustard
¼ tsp. sea salt
Freshly ground black pepper, to taste

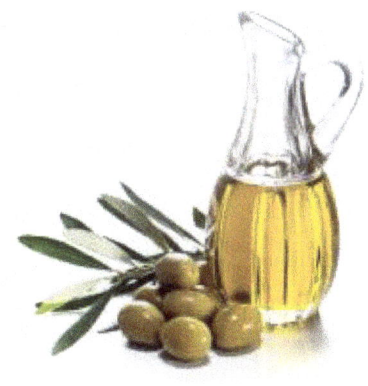

Instructions
Whisk all ingredients together until blended.
For the best flavor,
let it sit for 10-15 minutes before serving.

Vinaigrette Dressing
⅓ cup low-sodium chicken broth
1 Tbsp. chopped fresh basil
1 Tbsp. extra-virgin olive oil
1 Tbsp. fresh lemon juice
1 garlic clove, minced
1 tsp. Dijon mustard
Ground black pepper, to taste

Instructions
Place all ingredients except the olive oil in a blender or food processor.

Pulse until combined.

With the motor running, slowly drizzle in the olive oil in a thin stream, scraping down the sides as needed, until smooth, creamy, and bright green.

Parsley Basil Dressing
1 cup packed flat-leaf parsley (lower stems removed; about 1 small bunch)

½ cup loosely packed fresh basil leaves

1 garlic clove, crushed

1 Tbsp. fresh lemon juice

Salt and ground black pepper, to taste

¼ cup extra-virgin olive oil

Instructions
Combine all ingredients except the olive oil in a food processor
and pulse until roughly blended.

Slowly drizzle in the olive oil while blending,
scraping down the sides as needed,
until smooth, creamy, and bright green.

Herb Dressing
1 Tbsp. extra-virgin olive oil

2 Tbsp. flaxseed oil (optional)

Juice of 1 lemon

2 tsp. red wine vinegar

2 garlic cloves, minced

1 tsp. dried oregano

½ tsp. dried basil

Salt and freshly ground black pepper, to taste

Instructions
Whisk all ingredients together in a small bowl until well blended

Serve immediately or ref.rigerate for up to 3 days.

Natural, existing in or caused by nature; not made or caused by humankind.

Example: "Carrots contain a natural antiseptic that fights bacteria."

Breast cancer treatment can leave you feeling less than 100%, and your appetite may not be what it usually is. However, it's more important than ever to focus on the foods you're putting into your body.

"A balanced diet supports a healthy immune system, maintains electrolytes and muscle mass," Taylor says. "It also provides energy and helps combat the fatigue that is so often associated with cancer treatment." Aim to eat five to six small meals per day, as they're less likely to trigger uncomfortable side effects like nausea, vomiting, or diarrhea. Smaller meals also maximize your body's ability to absorb nutrients.

California Salad

Sunny California skies and balmy weather mean fresh produce year-round, like tomatoes and avocado that shine in this vibrant salad. Seasoned chicken adds plenty of savory flavor and keeps you feeling satisfied longer.

Ingredients

2 skinless, boneless chicken breasts
½ tsp. chili powder (mild or hot)
½ tsp. garlic powder
1 tsp. grated fresh ginger
¼ tsp. salt
¼ tsp. freshly ground black pepper
1 Tbsp. extra-virgin olive oil (first cold-pressed, organic)
6 cups mixed organic greens (e.g., baby kale, spinach, arugula)
2 Tbsp. fresh lemon juice
2 garlic cloves, minced
1 cup cherry tomatoes, halved
1 cup artichokes, chopped
½ cup onion (red, white, or green, your choice), sliced
2 ripe avocados, sliced

Instructions

Cook the Chicken
Season chicken with chili powder, garlic powder, ginger, salt, and pepper.

Heat a large skillet over high heat, then add the olive oil.

Add chicken, reduce the heat to medium, and cook 7-8 minutes, turning once or twice, until cooked through and no longer pink in the center.

Transfer chicken to a cutting board and let rest for 5 minutes before slicing.

Prepare the Dressing Base
In the same skillet, add lemon juice and garlic.

Stir well, scraping up any browned bits, then set aside.

Assemble the Salad
Spread greens evenly on a platter.

Top with tomatoes, avocado, artichokes, onion, and the lemon-garlic mixture from the skillet.

Slice chicken and arrange over the salad.

Divide into portions and serve immediately.

Quick Tip: Short on time? Use leftover cooked chicken or even rotisserie chicken to create this salad in minutes.

Southwestern Fish Salad

YIELD: 4 SERVINGS

This savory steak salad with creamy lime dressing that clings to the leaves will soon be a regular on your lunch or dinner table. Leftover meat for additional salads can be stored for up to 3 days. You can make this salad quickly by using leftover prepared steak.

Ingredients

Arctic Char, Lake Trout, Mackerel, or Salmon
2 Garlic Cloves, minced
1 tsp.EVOO
½ tsp. Salt
1 tsp. Chili Powder
1/2 tsp. Ground Cumin
1/4 c Cilantro chopped
Pepper
Salad
8 oz. Romaine Lettuce, chopped
1 c. Mushrooms and Onions (recipe is on page 20)
¼ c. Cilantro Leaves
2 Tbsp. Jalapenos, chopped (Optional)
Zesty Line Dressing
1 Lime, zested and juiced (about 2 Tbsp.) 1 Tbsp. EVOO
1 tsp. Dijon Mustard

Instructions

For The Fish:

Heat a large skillet or grill over medium heat.
Rub fish with crushed garlic cloves, olive oil, salt, pepper, Chili powder, and cumin.
Transfer fish to skillet or grill and cook 12-15 minutes (or less if a thinner cut of fish, turning occasionally until the meat is pink in the center but not translucent.
Rest 5 minutes on a cutting board..

For the Salad Dressing:

Place the lime zest and juice in a bowl.

Add olive oil and mustard.

Whisk well

To Assemble:

In a bowl, add the romaine, grilled mushrooms and onions, cilantro, and jalapenos.
Pour the dressing over the vegetables.
Top with the fish.
Serve immediately.

Chopped Salad

YIELD: 4 SERVINGS

Chopped salad is available at many places, but it can really add calories and fat. Pre-prep the veggies so that they are ready when you are hungry. You will be so glad that you did.

Ingredients

6 C. romaine lettuce, chopped
2 C. baby spinach
12 Oz. cooked turkey breast, chopped
2 hard-boil eggs, peeled and chopped
1 medium avocado, chopped
½ medium cucumber, peeled and chopped
1 Tbsp. red onion, finely chopped
4 Tbsp. extra-virgin olive oil
½ Tsp. dijon mustard
2 Tbsp. fresh squeezed lemon
A pinch of salt and freshly ground black pepper

Put It Together

In a large bowl, add the chopped lettuce, baby spinach, turkey breast, avocado, cucumber, bacon, and onion.
In a small bowl, combine the olive oil, dijon mustard, cider vinegar, salt and pepper until lightly emulsified.
Drizzle dressing over the salad, and toss.

Serve Immediately

Rather than purchase deli meat, roast your own turkey breast. Season with salt, pepper, poultry seasoning, onion & garlic powder. Slice thin or dice. It can also be used as a roll-up.

Salad Niçoise

This recipe is a twist on the classic French salad. You can dress it up with other fresh vegetables, such as steamed cauliflower or broccoli, or keep it simple and traditional with tomatoes and green beans.

Ingredients

2 (5 oz.) cans chunky light tuna packed in extra-virgin olive oil, well drained
(or cook and flake a tuna fillet, Arctic char, or mackerel)
2 hard-boiled eggs, quartered
1 (15 oz.) jar artichoke hearts, well drained and coarsely chopped
1 ½ tbsp capers, drained (or to taste)
6 cups arugula
1 cup black olives, pitted and drained
1 pint cherry tomatoes
¼ red onion, very thinly sliced
2 cups fresh or frozen green beans, cooked according to package directions
¼ tsp salt
¼ tsp freshly ground black pepper

Herb Dressing

3 tbsp extra-virgin olive oil
2 tbsp flaxseed oil (optional)
Juice of 1 ½ lemons
2 cloves garlic, minced
1 tsp dried oregano (or 1 tbsp. fresh)
½ tsp dried basil (or 1tbsp. fresh)
Salt and freshly ground black pepper, to taste.

Instructions

In a small jar, combine all herb dressing ingredients and whisk well. Set aside.
In a medium bowl, combine the tuna, artichoke hearts, and capers.
Fold in a portion of the herb dressing to coat.
In a large bowl, make a bed of arugula.
Add the olives, tomatoes, onion, and green beans.
Spoon the tuna mixture evenly over the top.
Add the quartered hard-boiled eggs.
Drizzle with the desired amount of herb dressing and serve immediately.

Artichoke, Tomato & Cucumber Salad

A Light Salad For Any Meal

Fresh, simple, and packed with flavor. This salad makes a refreshing side dish or a healthy main course.

Ingredients

1 ripe tomato, diced

1 cup organic canned artichokes, sliced

1 small cucumber, sliced

1 Tbsp. fresh lemon juice

1 Tbsp. olive oil

½ tsp. black pepper

½ tsp. dried oregano

Instructions

Combine all ingredients in a bowl.

Toss gently and let sit for 5 minutes to allow the flavors to blend.

Serve immediately and enjoy.

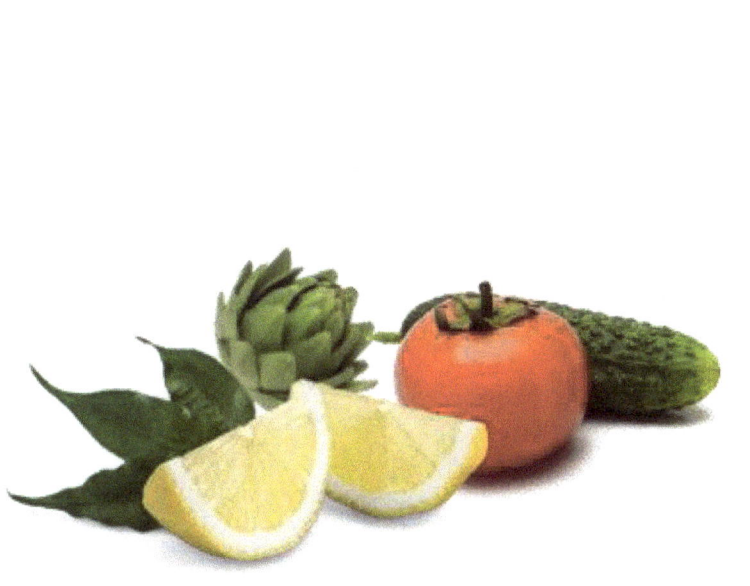

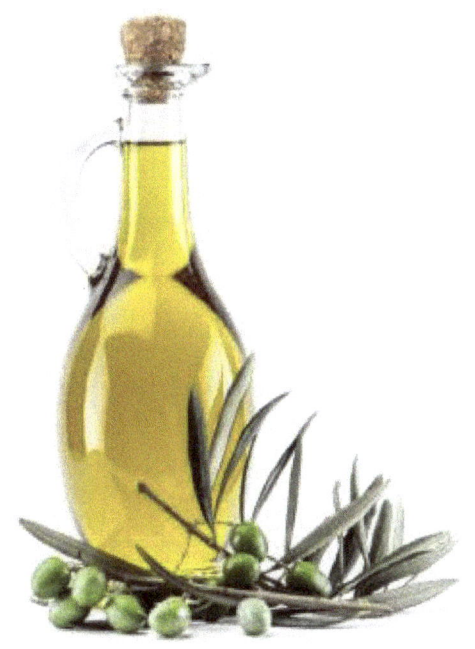

Nutrition Note

You've heard the phrase, *"An apple a day keeps the doctor away."*
Well, how about: *"Tomatoes each week keep your health at peak?"*
The National Institutes of Health (NIH) reviewed 72 human and animal studies and concluded that lycopene, a powerful compound found in tomatoes, has anticancer properties.
Lycopene helps prevent oxidative damage to DNA, lipids, and proteins, supports immune function, and even promotes the natural death of unhealthy cells, which can inhibit cancer cell growth.

Cabbage & Carrot Slaw With Lemon Dressing

A light, crunchy, and refreshing slaw that pairs perfectly with grilled meats, sandwiches, or as a healthy side dish.

Ingredients

2 cups shredded cabbage
1 medium carrot, grated
1 Tbsp. olive oil
1 Tbsp. fresh lemon juice
½ tsp. black pepper
½ tsp. garlic powder

Instructions

In a large bowl, combine all ingredients.
Toss well to coat evenly.

Let it sit for 10 minutes to allow flavors to blend.
Serve chilled or at room temperature.

Tip: For extra flavor, add a sprinkle of fresh parsley
or a dash of apple cider vinegar.

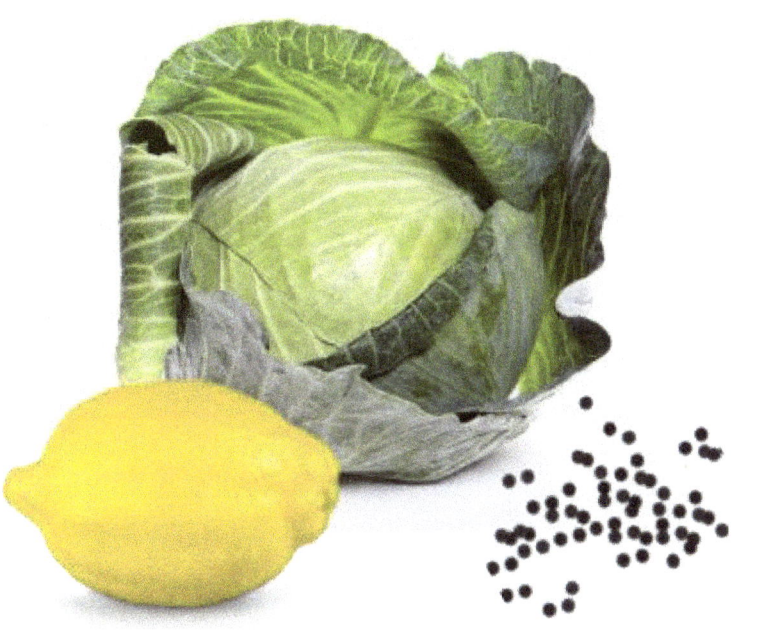
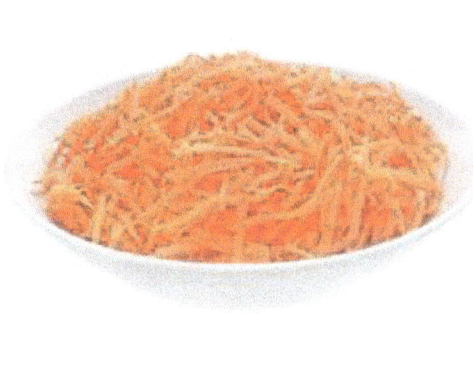

Chicken Pesto Salad

Pesto is simple to make and full of flavor. By blending basil, garlic, olive oil, and walnuts, you can create a delicious pesto sauce that transforms ordinary chicken salad into a gourmet dish. If you don't enjoy walnuts, pistachios are a great alternative. You can also experiment with almonds or cashews, just choose the nut you prefer. Remember, tree nuts provide more nutritional benefits than ground nuts.

Ingredients

12 oz bag broccoli slaw mix, chopped
2 cups diced cooked chicken *(baking chicken breasts in advance makes prep easier)*
1 cup fresh basil or baby arugula *(each provides a slightly different flavor)*
¼ cup walnuts *(or pistachios, almonds, etc.)*
3–4 Tbsp olive oil
1 Tbsp freshly grated Parmesan or Romano cheese
Salt and pepper, to taste
Sliced olives (optional)
Mixed greens or lettuce leaves

Instructions

Prepare the pesto by combining basil (or arugula), garlic, nuts, cheese (optional), salt, and pepper in a food processor.

Drizzle in the olive oil gradually while processing, scraping down the sides until smooth and blended to your desired consistency.

In a large bowl, mix the broccoli slaw, cooked chicken, and pesto until evenly coated.

Serve over mixed greens or use large lettuce leaves as wraps.

Top with sliced olives, if desired.

Spicy Chicken And Egg Salad

Like it spicy? *Adjust the heat to your taste, add more or less Tabasco, or kick it up a notch with red pepper flakes or fresh chili peppers.*

Ingredients

¼ cup homemade mayonnaise (see recipe below)
4 hard-boiled eggs, chopped
1 Tbsp. freshly squeezed lemon juice
½ tsp. Tabasco sauce *or* hot wing sauce (add more to taste)
¼ tsp. Himalayan salt *or* celery salt (preferred)
1 cup shredded cooked chicken
4 lettuce leaves
1 tomato, chopped

Instructions

In a medium bowl, combine the mayonnaise, lemon juice, Tabasco sauce, and salt.
Gently fold in the chopped eggs and shredded chicken.
Spoon the mixture into lettuce leaves and top with chopped tomato.
Serve immediately, or chill for 15 minutes for flavors to develop.

Homemade Mayonnaise

Ingredients

1 large egg (room temperature)
1 Tbsp. Dijon mustard
1 Tbsp. freshly squeezed lemon juice
¼ tsp. fine sea salt *or* celery salt
1 cup very light olive oil (the lighter the flavor, the better)

Instructions

Add all ingredients to a wide-mouth Mason jar.
Allow the oil to settle on top.
Place an immersion blender at the bottom of the jar and blend without moving until the mayonnaise begins to emulsify.
Slowly tilt and raise the blender to incorporate the remaining oil until smooth and creamy.
Transfer to an airtight container and refrigerate. Use within 2 weeks.

Put It Together

Place eggs in a large saucepan and cover with 1 inch of cool water.
Bring the water to a full boil (about 5-7 minutes). Remove from heat, cover, and let sit for 10 minutes.
Meanwhile, prepare a large bowl of ice water. Using a slotted spoon, transfer the eggs to the ice water and let them cool for a few minutes. Peel the eggs, chop them, and set aside.
In a medium bowl, whisk together the mayonnaise, lemon juice, hot sauce, and salt until smooth.
Fold in the chopped chicken and eggs until well combined.
To assemble the wraps, lay 2 pieces of lettuce on each wrap and top with half of the chopped tomatoes. Spoon half of the chicken-egg salad mixture over the lettuce and tomatoes. Roll tightly to close, slice in half if desired, and serve immediately

Curried Egg Salad

SERVES: 4

TOTAL TIME: 20 MIN

INGREDIENTS
8 large eggs
2 Tbsp organic mayonnaise
2 Tbsp low-fat Greek yogurt
1 tsp curry powder
Celery salt
White pepper

DIRECTIONS
Place the eggs in a saucepan and add enough water to cover.

Bring to a boil, turn the heat to simmer, cover, and cook 8
minutes.

Remove from heat, and with a slotted spoon, remove each egg
and place it into a bowl of ice water, gently cracking each one.
This makes peeling easier. Peel and coarsely chop.

In a medium bowl, combine the mayonnaise, yogurt, and curry powder.
Fold in the eggs and season with celery salt and pepper. Serve on top of
a salad with tomatoes, onion, cucumbers,
broccoli, and avocados.

Note: If you do not like curry, omit it and add 2 tsp mustard
and a dash of dill pickle juice.

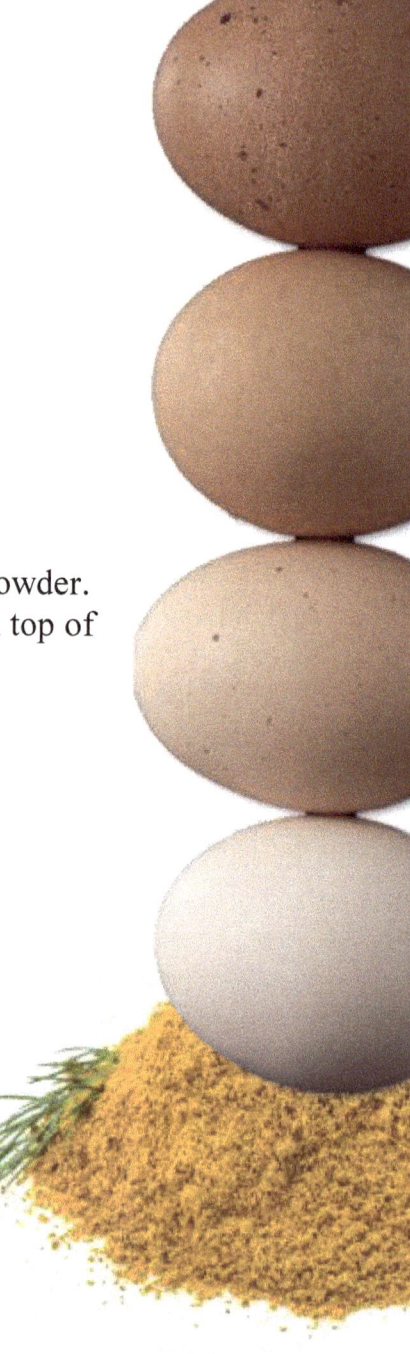

Tahini Chicken Salad

YIELD: 4 SERVINGS

Tahini is a rich paste made from ground sesame seeds, sometimes called sesame paste or sesame butter. Its flavor is amazing and pairs perfectly with chicken.

Ingredients

1 clove garlic, crushed

¼ cup tahini

Juice and zest of ½ lemon (or 1 Tbsp lemon, lime, or orange juice)

1 tsp tamari (gluten-free)

2 chicken breasts, cooked, boneless, skinless, and diced or shredded

At least 1 ½ cups raw or blanched green vegetables (e.g., 1-inch green beans, broccoli florets, chopped sugar snap peas, diced bell peppers, carrots, cauliflower, celery, artichokes, etc.)

1 cup grape tomatoes

¼ cup walnuts, crushed

¼ cup pitted black olives

8 to 12 large lettuce leaves

Instructions

Combine the tahini, lemon juice and zest, lime or orange juice, tamari, and 2 tablespoons of water in a food processor.

Process until smooth, scraping down the sides as necessary.

If the dressing is too thick or sticky, add more water, 1 tablespoon at a time.

Transfer the dressing to a medium bowl.

Add the chicken, green vegetables, tomatoes, walnuts, and olives. Toss gently to coat well.

Serve over lettuce leaves.

Indian Turkey Burger Salad

Using exotic Indian spices creates this flavorful turkey burger. Preparing the patties and sauce ahead of time ensures easy meal preparation. Use a meat thermometer to achieve perfect doneness.

Ingredients

Turkey Burgers

- 1 egg
- 1 lb lean ground turkey
- 2 Tbsp ground flaxseed
- ¼ cup green onion, chopped
- 1 Tbsp Dijon mustard
- 1 clove garlic, minced
- 1 Tbsp fresh chopped curry leaves (or cilantro)
- 1 Tbsp ginger, minced
- 1 tsp curry powder

Sauce

- ½ cup homemade mayonnaise
- ½ tsp curry powder
- 1 tsp fresh squeezed lemon juice
- 2 Tbsp minced fresh curry leaves (or cilantro)
- 2 drops vanilla stevia (optional)
- 1 cup light olive oil

Homemade Mayonnaise

- 1 whole egg
- 2 Tbsp. lemon juice
- ½ tsp Dijon mustard (or 1 tsp dry mustard powder)
- ¼ tsp salt
- ½ tsp onion powder
- ¼ tsp garlic powder
- ½ tsp cumin
- ¾ tsp salt
- ½ tsp pepper

Salad

- 4 cups arugula
- 2 cups sprouts (broccoli, pea, or alfalfa)
- 1 tomato, chopped
- 1 cucumber, diced

Instructions

Preheat grill or grill pan to medium heat.

In a large bowl, whisk the egg until lightly beaten.

Add the turkey, flaxseed, green onion, mustard, garlic, ginger, curry powder, cumin, salt, and pepper.

Mix gently with your hands.

Form into 4 equal patties.

Spray the grill or grill pan with high-heat cooking oil and cook the burgers until cooked through, about 5–6 minutes per side (internal temperature should reach 165°F / 74°C).

While the burgers are cooking, prepare the mayonnaise for the sauce.

Add all mayonnaise ingredients to a wide-mouth mason jar.

Allow the oil to rise to the top.

Place an immersion blender at the bottom of the jar and blend.

As the mayo emulsifies, slowly tilt the blender to incorporate the remaining oil.

Refrigerate any unused portion in an airtight container and use within two weeks.

Prepare the sauce:

In a small bowl, combine the mayonnaise, curry powder, lemon juice, cilantro, and stevia (if using).

Assemble the salads: make 4 beds with equal portions of arugula, tomato, and sprouts.

Top each salad with a turkey burger and drizzle with the sauce to taste.

Wraps

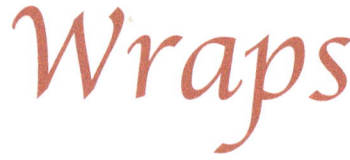

Wraps are a nutritious, low-carb option that provides essential vitamins and minerals without unnecessary carbohydrates. For those facing breast cancer, proper nutrition is especially important for maintaining strength and overall health.

The ingredients in these wraps not only supply vital nutrients but also contain cancer fighting properties that support healing and help the body defend against cancer cells. Eating smaller, more frequent meals throughout the day can also be easier to manage, particularly when coping with nausea or fatigue.

You will enjoy these tasty, nutritious wraps. So delicious and so easy to make.

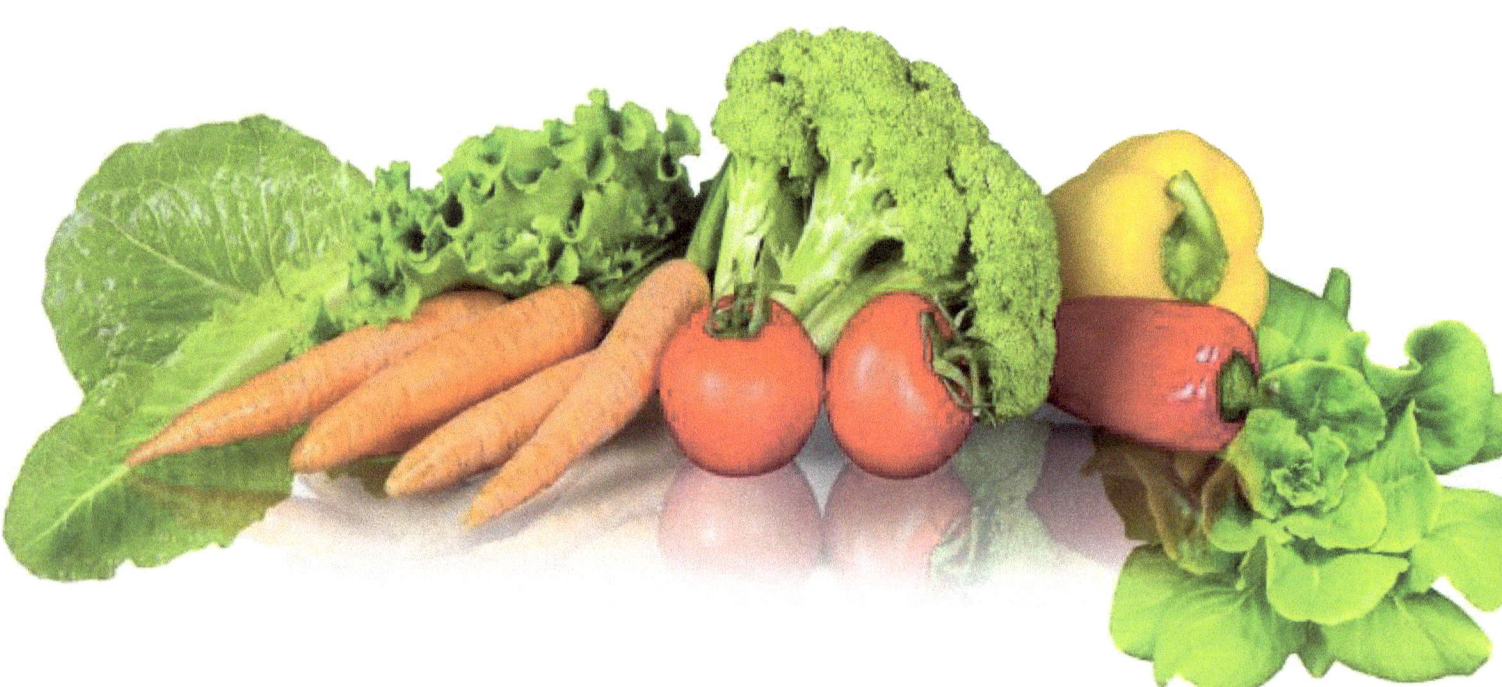

Cowboy Caviar

Yum!!

TOTAL TIME: 20 MINUTES
SERVINGS: 12

INGREDIENTS

3 roma tomatoes, seeds removed and diced
2 avocados, diced
⅓ cup diced red onion
1 (15 oz) can black beans, rinsed and drained
1 (15 oz) can kidney beans, rinsed and drained
1 ½ cups green beans, cut into ½-inch pieces
1 bell pepper, diced (any color)
1 jalapeno, seeds removed and finely diced *(omit if you don't like heat)*
1 cup mushrooms, diced
⅓ cup chopped fresh cilantro
1 can artichoke hearts, chopped
Tortilla chips, for serving

DRESSING

⅓ Cup Olive Oil
2 Tbsp fresh lime juice
2 tbsp red wine vinegar
15-20 drops lime stevia
½ tsp salt
½ tsp black pepper
1-2 cloves garlic, finely minced or grated

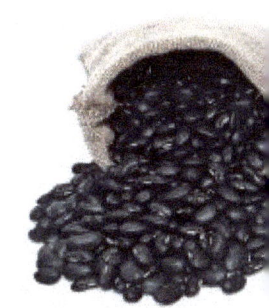

INSTRUCTIONS

Combine the tomatoes, avocado, red onion, black beans, kidney beans, mushrooms, green beans, bell pepper, jalapeño, cilantro, and artichoke hearts in a large bowl.
Stir well until evenly combined.
In a separate bowl, whisk together the olive oil, lime juice, red wine vinegar, stevia, salt, pepper, and garlic.
Pour the dressing over the salad ingredients and stir well to coat.
Refrigerate until ready to serve. if not serving immediately, stir again just before serving. Serve with tortilla chips or rolled up in lettuce leaves.

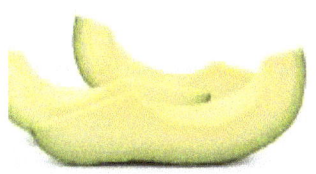

Turkey Wraps

YIELD: 2 SERVINGS

Choosing deli meat that is real, organic turkey is important. Aim to eat as cleanly as possible.

Ingredients

2 cups packed baby spinach or kale

¾ cup carrots

1 cucumber, peeled and finely chopped

2 tsp finely minced fresh ginger or fresh-squeezed lemon juice

12 thin slices of organic, gluten-free deli turkey

1–2 Hass avocados, peeled and mashed into a paste

Tip: *You can also roast your own organic turkey breast and slice it thinly.*

Instructions

Combine the spinach and carrots in a food processor.

Pulse until finely chopped but not pureed, scraping down the sides as needed.

Stir in the ginger or lemon juice.

Double up the turkey slices to create 6 turkey "wraps."

Spread equal amounts of avocado onto each wrap.

Spoon equal portions of the spinach-carrot mixture over the avocado, then top with cucumbers.

Roll the turkey wraps tightly.

Serve immediately.

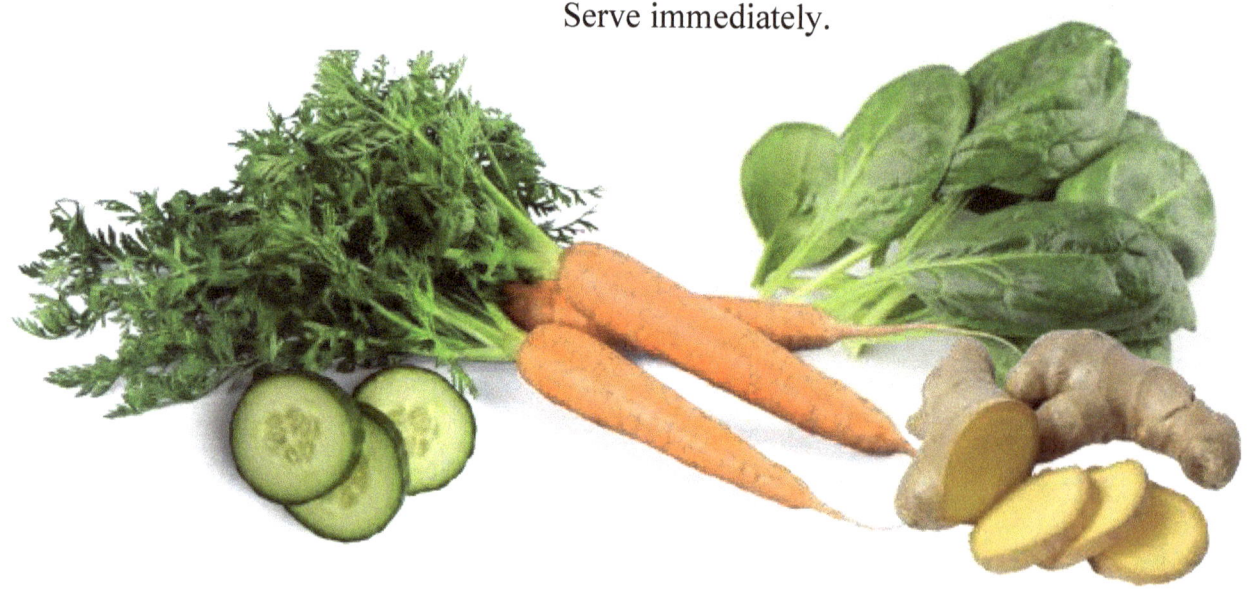

Chicken Artichoke Wraps

YIELD: 2-3 SERVINGS

Try these refreshing lettuce wraps packed with healthy fats from green olives, olive oil, and creamy avocado. Artichokes add a boost of antioxidants and provide an excellent source of dietary fiber, folate, and vitamins C and K.

Ingredients

½ cup celery, finely chopped

1 (15 oz) jar artichoke hearts in water, drained and chopped
½ cup pitted green olives (optional)

10 oz cooked chicken breast, diced small

1 avocado, sliced

1 Tbsp organic mayonnaise *(homemade works great too)*
½ tsp onion powder or ⅓ cup red onion, finely chopped

Celery salt, to taste

Romaine leaves, for wraps

Instructions

In a medium bowl, combine celery, artichokes, green olives, chicken, mayonnaise, and red onion (if using).

Season with celery salt and onion powder, adjusting to taste. Mix until well combined.

Spoon small portions of the mixture into romaine lettuce leaves.

Top each wrap with avocado slices. Fold or roll the leaves and serve immediately.

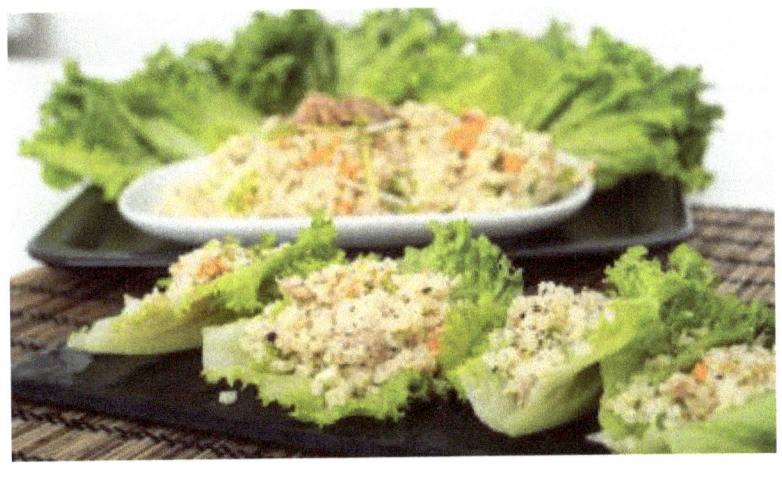

Tuna Wraps with Artichokes & Olives

YIELD: 2-3 SERVINGS

Tuna wrapped in crisp lettuce makes a fresh and healthy lunch. These wraps provide plenty of healthy fats from green olives, olive oil, and avocado slices. Artichokes are not only antioxidant- rich, but also a great source of dietary fiber, folate, and vitamins C and K. Fun fact: they also act as a natural flavor enhancer!

Ingredients

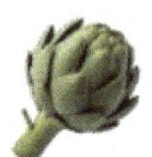

1 (15 oz.) jar marinated artichoke hearts, drained (reserve liquid)

½ cup pitted green olives, sliced

2 (5 oz.) cans chunk light tuna in extra-virgin olive oil, well-drained

1 tsp. extra-virgin olive oil

Salt and freshly ground black pepper, to taste

¼ tsp. onion powder

¼ tsp. garlic powder

½ avocado, sliced

1 cup grape tomatoes (½ diced, ½ quartered)

¼ cup nonfat Greek yogurt

Romaine or Bibb lettuce leaves, for wraps

Instructions

Slice the artichoke hearts and combine them with the olives and tomatoes in a medium bowl. Stir in the tuna.

In a separate bowl, whisk together the reserved artichoke liquid, Greek yogurt, and 1 tsp. olive oil. Season with salt, pepper, onion powder, and garlic powder.

Pour the dressing over the tuna mixture and toss gently to combine.

Spoon onto romaine or Bibb lettuce leaves, top with avocado slices, and serve immediately.

Easy Meat Roll Ups

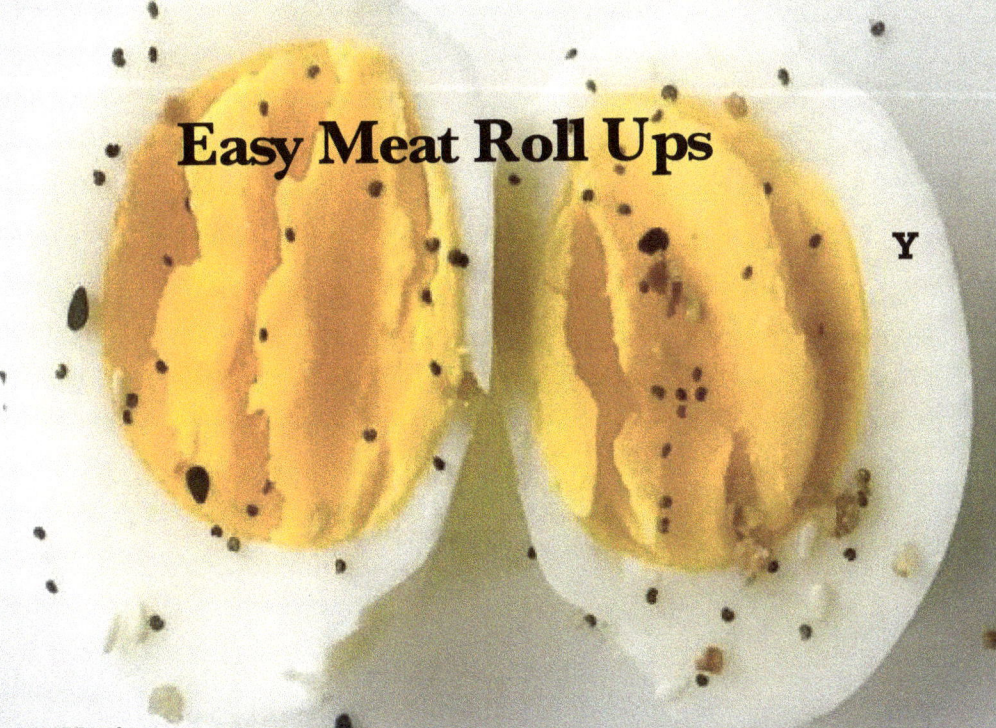

Y

Ingredients (Roll-Ups)

1 cup cabbage slaw (cabbage, thinly sliced; onion, finely chopped; carrot, grated)

6 oz. organic, minimally processed roast beef, chicken, or turkey (avoid deli meat, as it often contains additives and preservatives)

1 tomato, chopped

1 Tbsp. homemade mayonnaise (see recipe below)

Homemade Mayonnaise

Ingredients:

1 whole egg

½ tsp. Dijon mustard or 1 tsp. dry mustard powder (add more if desired)

2 Tbsp. lemon juice or vinegar

¼ tsp. salt

1 cup light, cold-pressed extra-virgin olive oil

Garlic and onion powder, to taste (optional, but adds great flavor)

Instructions:

Add all ingredients to a wide-mouth Mason jar, ending with the oil.

Place an immersion blender at the very bottom of the jar and blend.

As the mayonnaise emulsifies, slowly tilt the blender to incorporate the remaining oil until smooth and creamy.

Store in an airtight container in the refrigerator and use within 2 weeks.

Instructions (Roll-Ups)

In a medium bowl, combine the cabbage slaw, chopped tomato, and mayonnaise. Mix gently to coat evenly.

Lay out the slices of cooked meat.

Spread the veggie mixture over each slice, then roll up tightly to enclose the filling.

Veggies

Fruits And Vegetables Are Not Only Rich In vitamins, minerals, and fiber, but they also contain phytochemicals, powerful plant-based compounds that help fight cancer and lower the risk of its development.

Cruciferous vegetables such as broccoli, Brussels Sprouts, cabbage, cauliflower, and kale are especially noteworthy.
They contain phytochemicals called glucosinolates, which, during preparation and digestion, break down into biologically active compounds.

One of the most studied of these is sulforaphane, known for its ability to neutralize carcinogens, reduce inflammation, and promote the body's natural detoxification processes.

Several studies suggest that regular consumption of cruciferous vegetables may play a protective role by slowing the growth of cancer cells and even triggering apoptosis, or the programmed death of unhealthy cells. Including a variety of these vegetables in your diet can therefore contribute to long-term health and cancer prevention.

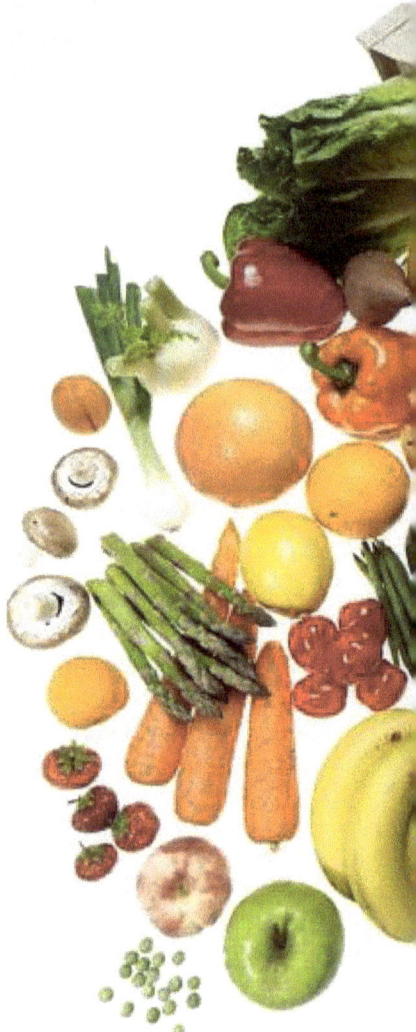

Zucchini and Spinach with Brown Butter

YIELD: 2 SERVINGS
(About 2 Cups Per Serving)

Browning butter gives this dish a wonderful nutty flavor that elevates simple vegetables. Fresh sage leaves turn mild and crispy when cooked in butter, adding a spark of flavor. If sage isn't your favorite, you can substitute it with diced tomato and fresh basil for a lighter twist.

Ingredients

2 Tbsp. unsalted butter

½ tsp. dried sage *or* fresh sage leaves, chopped (optional)
Alternative: 1 small tomato, diced, with fresh basil, chopped

1 small zucchini, thinly sliced

5 oz. baby spinach
⅓ tsp. salt

1 small onion, finely chopped (optional)

1 clove garlic, minced (optional)

Instructions

Place the butter in a large skillet over medium heat.

Cook until lightly browned and fragrant.

If using sage, add it and cook for 30 seconds.

For fresh sage leaves, cook until crisp.

Add the zucchini, baby spinach, and salt.

Toss well to coat with the butter.

Stir in onion and garlic if desired.

Cook just until the spinach wilts and the zucchini softens slightly.

Serve immediately.

Grilled Peppers And Onions

YIELD: 2 SERVINGS

(2 ½ C. Per Serving)

If you're a fan of grilled peppers and onions on a sausage sandwich, then you'll love this side dish. Leftovers are perfect in scrambled eggs or served alongside pork or beef, gently warmed.

Ingredients

1 Tbsp olive oil

2 onions, peeled and sliced

1 red, orange, or yellow bell pepper, seeded and sliced

½ tsp salt

Pinch of turmeric (optional)

1 tsp fresh rosemary leaves, chopped

¼ tsp pepper

2 cloves garlic, minced

Instructions

Heat a large skillet over medium-high heat.

Add the olive oil. Stir in the onions, peppers, salt, turmeric (if using), and rosemary.

Cook for 3–4 minutes, stirring often, until the peppers and onions soften.

Add the garlic and cook for another minute.

Serve immediately.

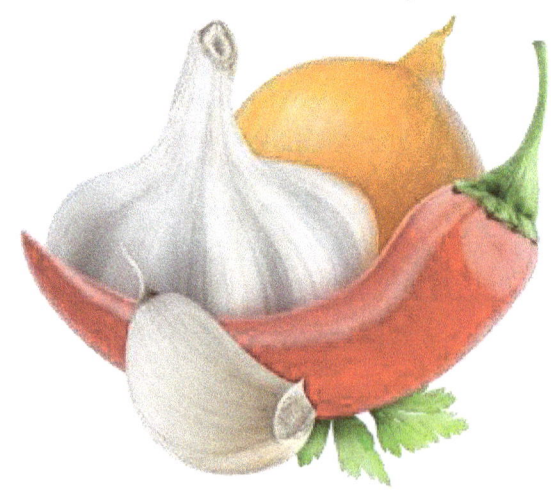

Roasted Turnips & Zucchini Medley

Full of flavor and nutrients to support your body's healing, this simple dish is delicious on its own or as a side with mackerel.

Ingredients

1–2 turnips, cubed

1 zucchini, sliced

1 Tbsp olive oil or black cumin oil

½ tsp black pepper

½ tsp saffron

½ tsp dried thyme

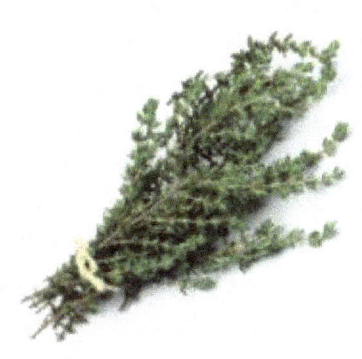

Instructions

Preheat oven to 400°F (200°C).

Toss the vegetables with olive oil and seasonings.

Spread on a baking sheet and roast for 25—30 minutes, until tender.

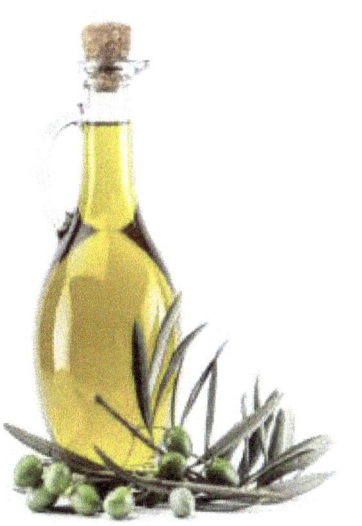

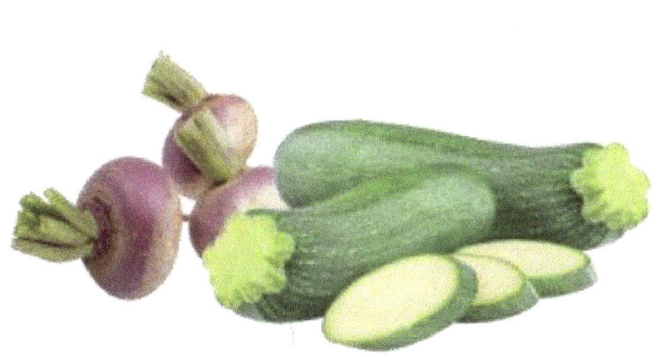

Zucchini & Bell Pepper Stir Fry

A quick, veggie–packed dish with a mild kick.

Ingredients

1 zucchini, sliced

1 bell pepper, sliced

½ onion, thinly sliced

1 Tbsp walnut or olive oil

½ tsp garlic powder

¼ tsp smoked paprika

¼ tsp black pepper

¼ tsp celery salt

Instructions

Heat the oil in a pan over medium heat.

Sauté the onion for 2 minutes, then add the zucchini and bell pepper.

Add the garlic powder, paprika, celery salt, and black pepper.

Cook until tender-crisp and serve warm.

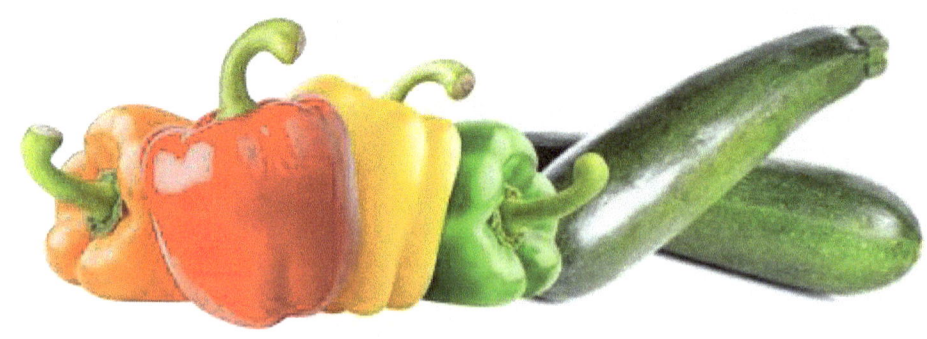

Pumpkin with Leeks and Pomegranate

A delicious, soft, and flavorful dish.

Ingredients

2 cups sugar pumpkin, diced
1 leek, thinly sliced
1 Tbsp ghee or walnut oil
2 cloves garlic, minced
Seeds from 1 pomegranate
½ tsp black pepper
Salt, to taste
½ tsp dried oregano

Instructions

Preparing the Pumpkin *(optional prep step)*:

The easiest way to prepare a pumpkin or butternut squash is to preheat your oven to 350°F. Pierce the pumpkin in several places, then place it on a parchment-lined baking sheet. Bake until it softens slightly, about 20—40 minutes, just enough so that you can press the skin with your finger. Do not overcook; this step only makes it easier to cut, peel, and dice. You can do this a day ahead, peeling and dicing once the pumpkin has cooled.

Cooking the Dish:

- Preheat the oven to 425°F and set an oven rack to the lowest position.
- Line a large, rimmed baking sheet with high-heat-resistant parchment paper.
- In a saucepan over medium heat, warm the ghee or walnut oil.
- Add the sliced leek and minced garlic and sauté until soft, about 5 minutes.
- In a large bowl, combine the diced pumpkin with the cooked leeks and garlic.
- Add oregano, salt, pepper, and a little more oil if needed, stirring until the pumpkin is well coated.
- Spread the pumpkin mixture in a single layer on the prepared baking sheet.
- Bake for about 30 minutes, tossing halfway through, until the pumpkin is tender.
- Garnish with fresh pomegranate seeds and serve immediately.

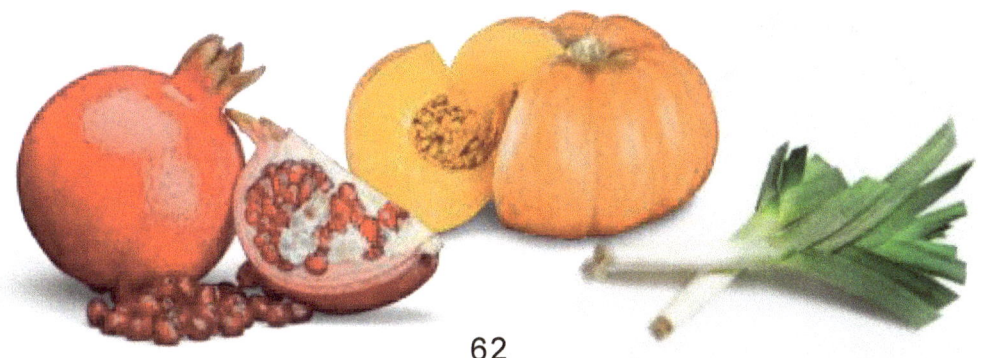

White Button Mushrooms

White button mushrooms are the most common type of mushroom consumed in the United States. They are a low-calorie, low-cholesterol, low-sodium food with a high fiber and protein content. Lisa Yee, MD, said they also offer a wide range of healthy ingredients, including vitamins, such as thiamin and niacin; minerals, such as iron, magnesium, manganese, zinc and selenium; and powerful antioxidants.

Most studies demonstrating the inverse relationship with white button mushroom consumption and breast cancer risk have been conducted in Asian countries, where their consumption is higher.

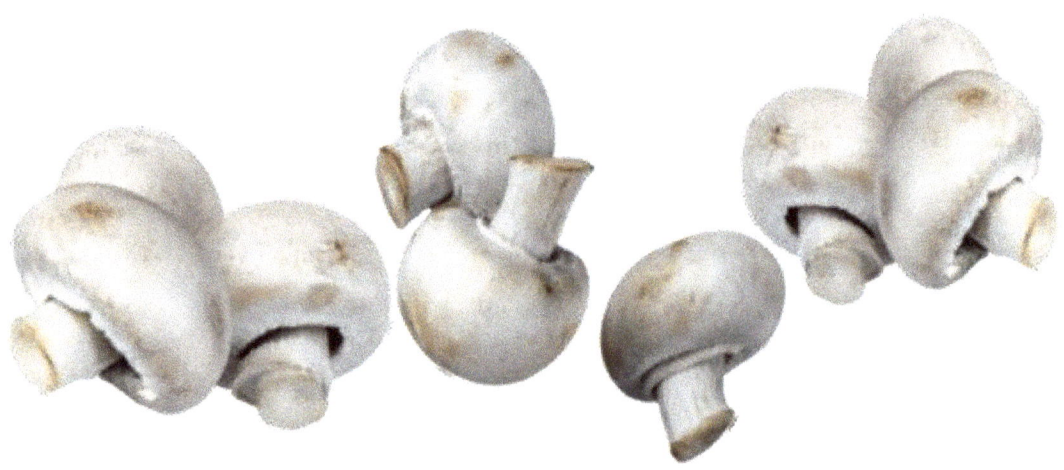

Chemicals in mushrooms have been found to slow the production of estrogen, as well as DHT. The intake of mushrooms has also been found to reduce one type of negative regulation of immune function. By the latter mechanism, white button mushroom intake is thought to improve our immune function to fight cancer.

Stuffed Pumpkin with Caramelized Onions, Mushrooms, Garlic, and Kale

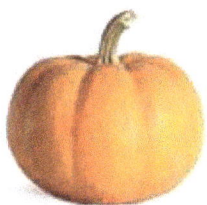

Ingredients

1 medium pumpkin (small enough to stuff)
2 Tbsp olive oil
1 large onion, thinly sliced
1 cup mushrooms, sliced *(cremini or shiitake work well)*
3 cloves garlic, minced
2 cups kale, chopped
½ tsp ground turmeric *(for warmth and color)*
½ tsp ground cumin *(earthy flavor)*
½ tsp ground coriander *(bright, citrusy undertone)*
¼ tsp cinnamon *(for a hint of sweetness)*
½ tsp ground ginger *(adds a little kick)*
Salt and pepper, to taste
Fresh herbs for garnish *(optional: parsley or thyme)*

Instructions

1. Preheat the oven to 375°F (190°C).
2. Slice off the top of the pumpkin (like a lid) and scoop out the seeds and pulp.
3. Rub the inside of the pumpkin with a little olive oil, salt, and pepper.
4. Place the pumpkin (with its lid) on a baking sheet a nd roast for 30—40 minutes, or until tender but firm, soft enough to eat but still holding its shape.
5. While the pumpkin is roasting, heat 1 Tbsp olive oil in a pan over medium heat. Add the sliced onion and cook slowly for about 15 minutes, stirring occasionally, until golden and caramelized.
6. Add the sliced mushrooms to the pan and cook for 5 minutes, until softened and browned.
7. Stir in the garlic and cook for 1—2 minutes. Add the kale and cook for another 2—3 minutes, until wilted.
8. Sprinkle in the turmeric, cumin, coriander, cinnamon, and ginger. Mix well and adjust seasoning with salt and pepper.
1. Once the pumpkin is roasted, carefully stuff it with the onion, mushroom, garlic, and kale mixture.
2. Top with fresh herbs, if desired, and return the stuffed pumpkin to the oven for an additional 10–15 minutes to let the flavors meld.
3. Carefully slice and serve, with a side salad if desired.

Cruciferous Veggies

Surgeon Marsha Nelson, MD, of the Valley Health Breast Center, emphasizes the importance of a healthy diet in reducing the risk of breast cancer.

Eating well is one of the most powerful steps you can take to lower your breast cancer risk. Unfortunately, most Americans follow the "Standard American Diet" (SAD—appropriately named), which is typically high in animal products and processed foods. By increasing your intake of fruits and vegetables to at least five servings a day, you can not only reduce your risk of developing breast cancer but also improve survival outcomes for those already diagnosed.

Cruciferous vegetables, such as broccoli, cauliflower, collards, cabbage, and kale are especially valuable. For example, studies have shown that women taking tamoxifen who included at least one serving of cruciferous vegetables among their five daily servings of fruits and vegetables cut their risk of cancer recurrence by as much as half.

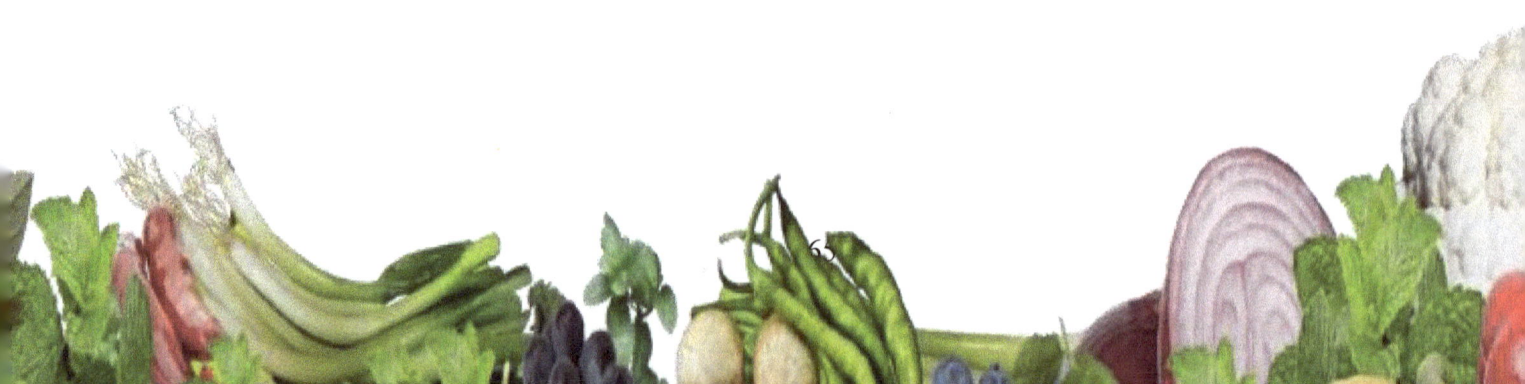

Garlic Broccoli

YIELD: 2 SERVINGS
(About 2 Cups Per Serving)

Garlic lovers will enjoy this savory yet light side dish. There's no need to steam the broccoli first; covering the pan allows the natural water content to cook the broccoli through.

Ingredients

1 Tbsp extra virgin olive oil (EVOO)

4 cups broccoli, cut into florets

4 garlic cloves, minced

¼ tsp salt

¼ tsp crushed red pepper flakes

1 small onion, thinly sliced *(or substitute a leek)*

Instructions

Heat a large skillet over medium heat.

Add the olive oil and onion (or leek) and cook for 3 minutes.

Stir in the broccoli, garlic, salt, and red pepper flakes.

Cook for 2 minutes, stirring often, until the garlic becomes fragrant.

Reduce the heat to low, cover, and cook for 2–3 minutes, until the broccoli is tender and cooked through.

Serve immediately.

Grilled Mushrooms and Onions

YIELD: 2 SERVINGS
(About 2 ½ Cups Per Serving)

If you're a fan of grilled mushrooms and onions, you'll love this savory side dish. Leftovers are perfect in scrambled eggs or served alongside chicken or fish, gently warmed.

Ingredients

2 Tbsp olive oil
2 onions, peeled and sliced
Mushrooms, sliced *(any variety works well)*
½ tsp salt
Pinch of turmeric
1 tsp fresh parsley, chopped
¼ tsp pepper
2 cloves garlic, minced

Instructions

Heat a large skillet over medium-high heat.
Add the olive oil.
Stir in the onions, mushrooms, salt, turmeric, and parsley.
Cook for 5–8 minutes, stirring often, until the mushrooms and onions soften.
Add the garlic and cook for 1 more minute.
Serve immediately.

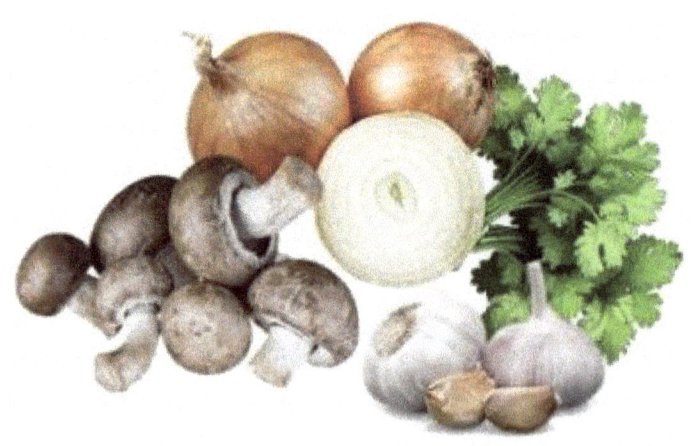

Broccoli with Garlic, & Red Pepper

YIELD: 2 SERVINGS
(About 2 Cups Per Serving)

I love garlic, and I love broccoli, and together they make an amazing combination. Red chili peppers of the genus Capsicum are a popular spice worldwide and contain capsicin. Research has shown that capsaicin reduced the volume of breast tumors in mice by 50% without noticeable side effects and suppressed the progression of preneoplastic breast lesions by 80%.

Ingredients

4 cups broccoli, cut into florets

4 garlic cloves, minced (or use jarred garlic to save time) ¼ tsp organic onion salt

¼ tsp crushed red pepper flakes *(optional)*

1 small onion, thinly sliced

Instructions

Heat a large skillet over medium heat.

Add a small amount of oil. Once hot, add the onion and cook for about 3 minutes, or until it begins to soften and caramelize. Stir in the garlic.

Add the broccoli, onion salt, and red pepper flakes.

Cook for 2 minutes, stirring often, until the garlic becomes fragrant.

Reduce the heat to low, cover, and cook for 2—3 minutes, until the broccoli is tender and cooked through.

Remove the cover and cook for 1 additional minute.

Serve immediately.

Lemony Green Beans With Crushed Walnuts

YIELD: 2 SERVINGS
(About 1 ½ Cups Per Serving)

Lemon and green beans bring a bright, spring-like flavor to this zesty dish that's elegant enough for evening entertaining. Short on time during the week? Trim and blanch the green beans in boiling water for 3 minutes, then place them in an ice bath to stop the cooking process. This will also keep them vibrant green. For convenience, zest and juice the lemon and crush the walnuts in advance; both can be stored in the refrigerator for up to 24 hours.

Ingredients

2 Tbsp olive oil
1 lb green beans, trimmed
1 lemon, zested and juiced
¼ cup walnuts, crushed
Celery salt, to taste

Instructions

Heat a large skillet over medium-high heat.
Add the olive oil, green beans, and lemon zest.
Toss well and cook for 2—3 minutes, until the beans are crisp-tender.
Reduce the heat to low and cook an additional 2—3 minutes, until the beans are cooked through but still have a slight snap.
Add the lemon juice and cook for 1 minute more, uncovered, to allow the juice to reduce slightly.
Add the walnuts and toss to combine. Serve immediately.

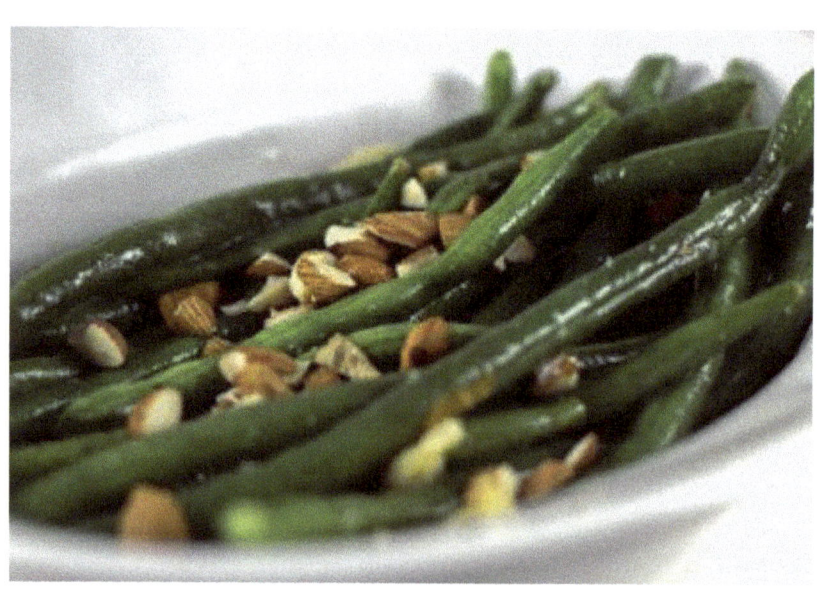

Mustard Greens with Tangy Dijon Glaze

YIELD: 2 SERVINGS

Tangy Dijon mustard makes a flavorful glaze for this simple spring vegetable dish. When shopping for mustard greens, look for baby greens, they're more tender, but always choose the freshest bunch you can find.

Ingredients

1 Tbsp. ghee

1 lb. mustard greens, trimmed

1 Tbsp. Dijon mustard

2 garlic cloves, minced

1 lb. mushrooms, sliced

1 onion, quartered and thinly sliced

½ tsp. stevia *or* 8–12 drops liquid stevia

½ tsp. celery salt

¼ tsp. black pepper

Instructions

Heat a large skillet over medium heat. Add the ghee.

Add the onion and cook for 1–2 minutes, stirring often, until it begins to brown.

Reduce the heat to low and add the mustard, garlic, stevia, and 2 Tbsp. water.

Sprinkle with celery salt and pepper.

Add the mushrooms and mustard greens. Cover and cook for 1–2 minutes, until the greens are wilted and tender.

Serve immediately.

Zucchini, Carrots And Spinach With Ghee

YIELD: 2 SERVINGS

Browning ghee gives this dish a rich, nutty flavor that transforms simple vegetables into something special. Fresh sage leaves become mild and crispy when cooked in ghee, adding a burst of flavor and texture.

Ingredients

1 Tbsp. organic ghee

½ tsp. dried sage *or* 4–6 fresh sage leaves, chopped (optional)

1 small zucchini, thinly sliced

5 oz. baby spinach

1 carrot, grated

½ tsp. salt

¼ tsp. black pepper

Instructions

- Place the ghee in a large skillet over medium heat.

- If using sage, add it and cook for 30 seconds. For fresh sage leaves, cook until crisp.

- Add the zucchini, spinach, carrot, salt, and pepper.

- Toss well to coat the vegetables evenly in the ghee.

- Cook just until the spinach wilts and the zucchini is tender-crisp.

- Serve immediately.

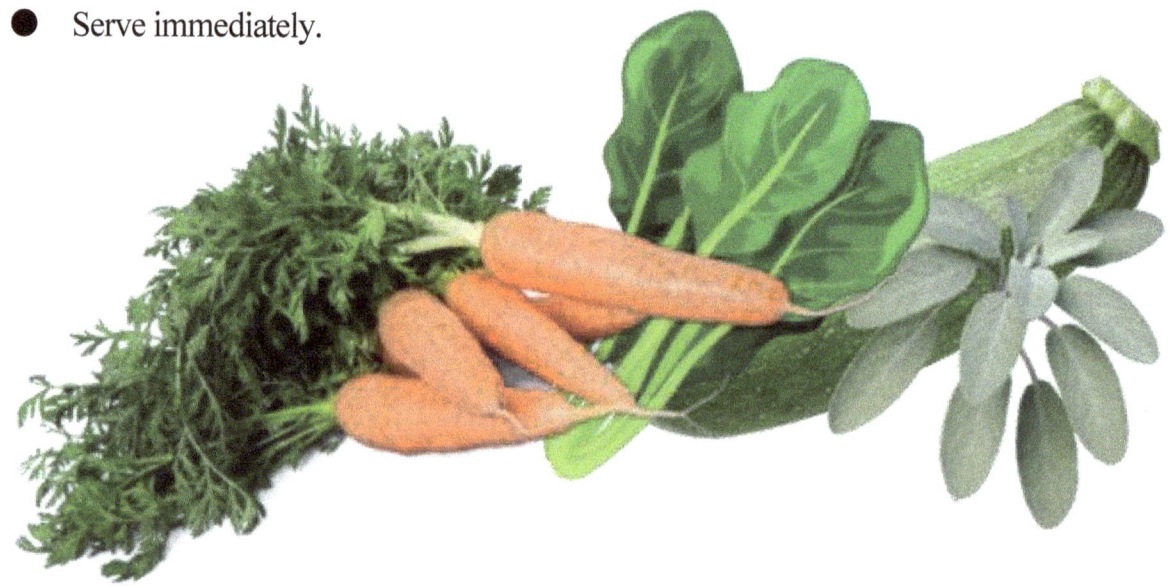

Bok Choy With Ginger

YIELD: 2 SERVINGS

Bok choy belongs to the same family as kale and broccoli. Many grocery stores carry it, but if yours doesn't, you can substitute the same amount of kale or broccoli. Just be sure to slice the kale or cut the broccoli into florets before cooking.

Ingredients

1 tsp. coconut oil

4 tsp. fresh ginger, minced

4 garlic cloves, minced

1 lb. bok choy, thinly sliced

¼ tsp. salt

1 Tbsp. ghee (preferably grass-fed)

1 lime, zested and juiced

1 Tbsp. fresh curry paste *or* 1 tsp. curry powder

Instructions

● Heat a large stockpot over medium heat.

● Add the coconut oil, ginger, garlic, and curry. Cook for about 1 minute, until fragrant.

● Add the bok choy and salt. Cook for 2–3 minutes more, stirring often.

● Stir in the ghee, lime zest, and lime juice. Toss well to combine.

● Serve immediately.

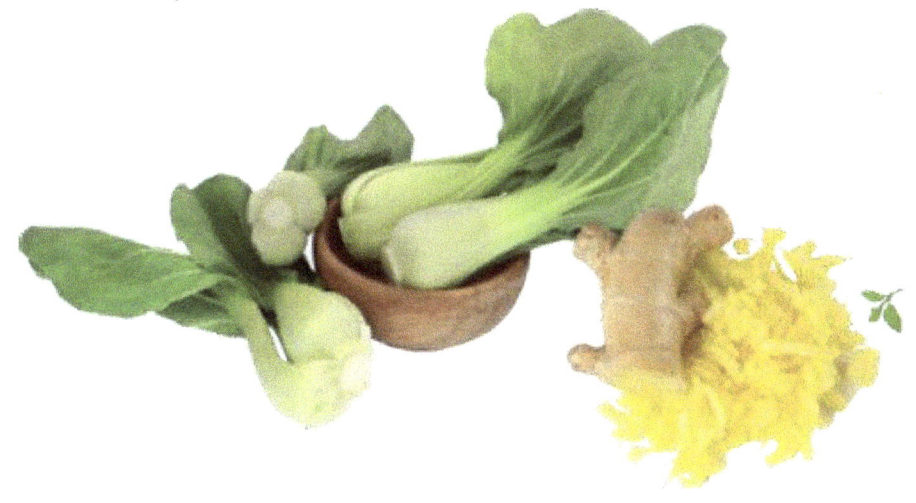

Sesame Spinach

YIELD: 2 SERVINGS

Sesame and tamari make a perfect match for this nutrient-packed superfood. spinach is rich in folate, fiber, and vitamin a, making this dish both wholesome and delicious. Serve it alongside salmon, grilled beef, or tofu for a satisfying, balanced meal.

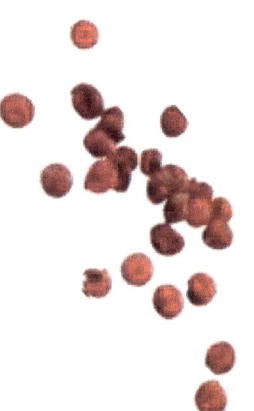

INGREDIENTS

1 tbsp. coconut oil

1 lb. baby spinach

1 tbsp. bragg's liquid aminos (or tamari/soy sauce)

1 tbsp. sesame seeds

½ tsp. himalayan salt

¼ tsp. freshly ground black pepper

instructions

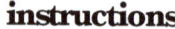

Heat a large stockpot or wok over high heat. add the coconut oil.

Add the spinach and press down gently with a small lid or spatula until wilted, about 1–2 minutes.

Reduce the heat to low. stir in the liquid aminos, sesame seeds, salt, and pepper. toss well to coat.

Serve immediately, warm.

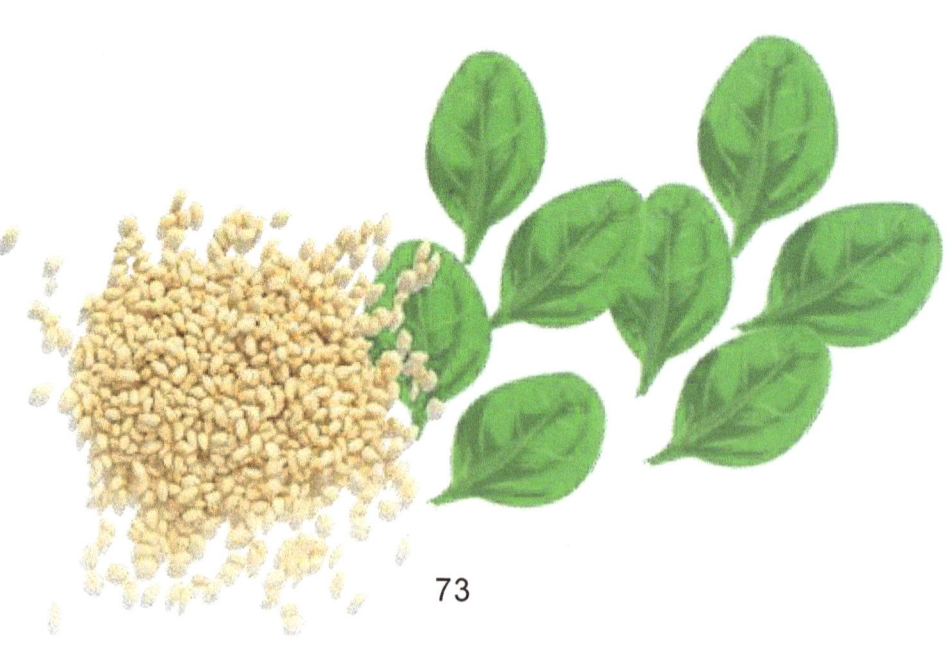

Broccoli with Garlic & Carrots

YIELD: 2 SERVINGS
(About 2 Cups PerServing)

Garlic lovers will enjoy this savory yet light broccoli side dish. The natural water in the vegetables creates gentle steam as they cook, so there's no need to pre-steam the broccoli. the result is tender-crisp florets with a garlicky punch and a hint of heat.

Ingredients

1 cup grated carrots

1 tbsp. olive oil or ghee
4 cups of broccoli florets

4 garlic cloves, minced

1 small onion, thinly sliced
¼ tsp. salt

¼ tsp. crushed red pepper flakes

Fresh lemon juice (optional, for brightness)

Instructions:

Heat a large skillet over medium heat. add the olive oil (or ghee) and onion. cook for about 3 minutes, until softened.

Add the broccoli, carrots, garlic, salt, and red pepper flakes.

Cook for 2 minutes, stirring often, until the garlic becomes fragrant.

Reduce the heat to low, cover, and cook for 2—3 minutes more, until the broccoli is tender but still vibrant green.

Remove from heat, drizzle with a squeeze of fresh lemon juice if desired, and serve immediately.

Broccoli Almondine

Crunchy almonds add texture and healthy fats to this quick and flavorful side dish. Smoked paprika and fresh lemon bring brightness and depth. If you can't find slivered almonds, simply chop whole almonds with a knife or mini-chopper.

Ingredients

1 Tbsp. organic ghee

¼ tsp. salt

1 bunch broccoli, cut into florets (about 4 cups)

½ lemon, zested and juiced

½ tsp. smoked paprika

¼ cup almonds, slivered or chopped

Instructions

Heat a large skillet over medium heat. Add the ghee, broccoli, paprika, salt, and lemon zest.
Cook for 1–2 minutes, stirring, until the broccoli begins to brown slightly.
Cover the skillet, reduce the heat to low, and cook for another 2 minutes, until broccoli is tender but still vibrant green.
Remove the lid, add lemon juice and almonds, and toss well.
Serve immediately as a fresh, crunchy side dish.

Variation

Green Beans Almondine: Substitute green beans for broccoli. Blanch the beans for 2–3 minutes before sautéing to keep them crisp-tender.
Add a pinch of red pepper flakes for a little heat.
Sprinkle with fresh parsley before serving for extra color and freshness.

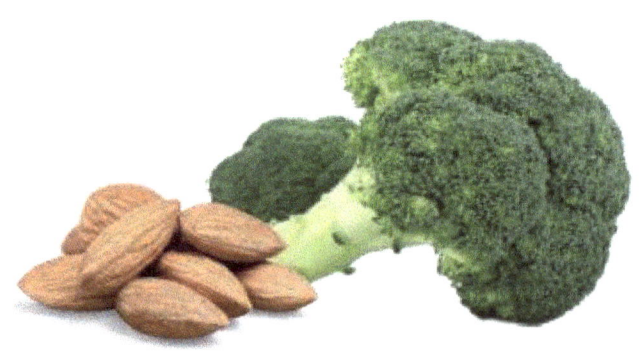

7-Ingredient Vegan Stuffed Mushrooms

COOK TIME: 1 HOUR

Ingredients

½ cup black rice (or substitute wild or brown rice)
1 scant cup vegetable stock
1 (10-ounce) package baby portobello or white button mushrooms*
¼ cup vegan Parmesan cheese *(plus more for topping; or*
Substitute regular Parmesan if not dairy-free)
¼ cup raw walnuts, crushed
1 ½ tsp finely minced garlic
1 ½ Tbsp olive oil (plus more for drizzling or coating)

Instructions

Preheat oven to 350°F (176°C). Rinse the rice in a fine-mesh strainer.
Bring the vegetable stock to a boil in a small saucepan, then add the rice. Lower the heat, cover, and cook until the liquid is completely absorbed—30 to 45 minutes. Taste for doneness. Cook longer if you prefer softer rice; for a firmer bite, check around the 25-minute mark.
While the rice is cooking, place the walnuts on a baking sheet and toast them in the oven for 5 minutes. Set aside.
Clean the mushrooms by brushing off dirt with a damp towel. Remove the stems. Brush or spray the caps with olive oil and set aside.
Prepare the Parmesan cheese (if making from scratch) and set aside.
Once the rice is cooked, fluff with a fork, then stir in the vegan Parmesan, toasted walnuts, minced garlic, and olive oil. Taste and adjust seasonings as needed. I added a pinch of salt, pepper, and a little extra Parmesan.
Bake the mushroom caps (without filling) on a baking sheet for 10 minutes to soften. Remove from the oven and fill each mushroom generously with the rice mixture. (You will have some leftover filling.) Top with additional vegan Parmesan and bake for another 15-18 minutes, or until the mushrooms are tender and the Parmesan is golden brown.

Baking the mushrooms first prevents the rice from becoming too crisp.
Serve immediately.
Tip: Dust your serving plate with vegan Parmesan so the bottoms of the mushrooms pick up extra flavor.

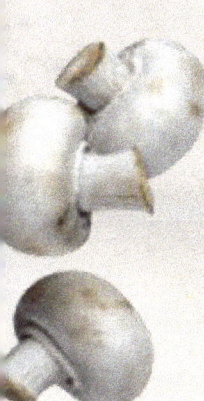

Protein

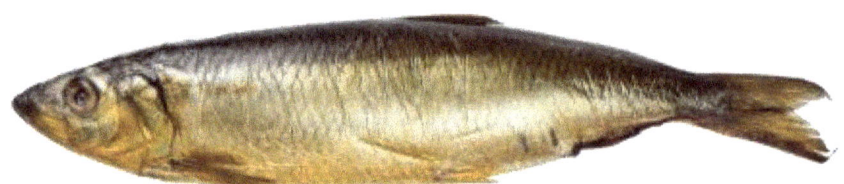

Proteins are large, complex molecules that perform most of the essential functions in our cells, tissues, and organs. They are made up of smaller building blocks called amino acids, which are often referred to as the "building blocks of life." Protein is critical for body maintenance, growth, and repair, and it also helps maintain lean body mass and muscle strength. Beyond muscle health, proteins play a vital role in producing enzymes and hormones, supporting immune function, and carrying oxygen throughout the body.

Everyone's protein needs are different, but during cancer treatment, the body requires even more protein. This is because protein helps the body repair tissues damaged by treatment, supports the immune system, and combats treatment-related muscle loss and fatigue.

A good rule of thumb:

- If you are eating regular portion sizes, aim to include protein three to four times per day.

- If you are eating smaller-than-usual portions, try to include protein four to five times per day to meet your needs.

- Great sources of protein include lean meats, poultry, fish, eggs, dairy products, beans, lentils, soy products, nuts, and seeds. Combining plant and animal sources can help ensure you're getting a full spectrum of essential amino acids.

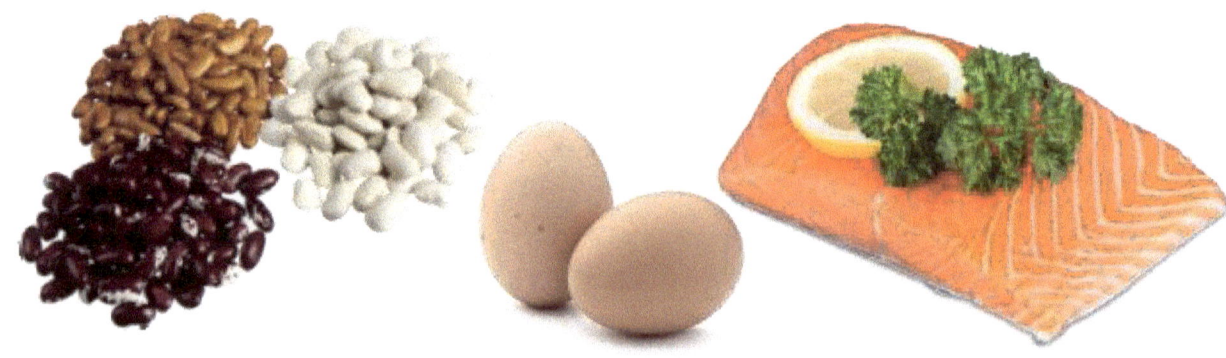

Easy Roasted Herb Chicken

Juicy, herb-roasted chicken baked on a bed of fresh vegetables makes for an easy, flavorful, and nutrient-packed dinner. The combination of basil, rosemary, and parsley (or cilantro), gives this dish a bright, aromatic finish.

Ingredients

4 cups broccoli florets *or* bok choy (chopped)
2 Tbsp. extra-virgin olive oil
2 Tbsp. fresh basil, chopped
¼ cup fresh parsley *or* cilantro, chopped
1 Tbsp. fresh rosemary, chopped
½ tsp. onion powder
½ tsp. garlic powder
¼ tsp. celery salt
4 chicken breasts, bone-in, skin-on

Instructions

Preheat the oven to 400°F (200°C). Line a baking sheet with aluminum foil.
Arrange the broccoli (or bok choy) in the center of the tray. Place the chicken breasts on top of the vegetables.
In a small bowl, whisk together the olive oil, basil, rosemary, parsley (or cilantro), onion powder, garlic powder, and celery salt.
Brush the herb oil evenly over the chicken, making sure to coat the skin well.

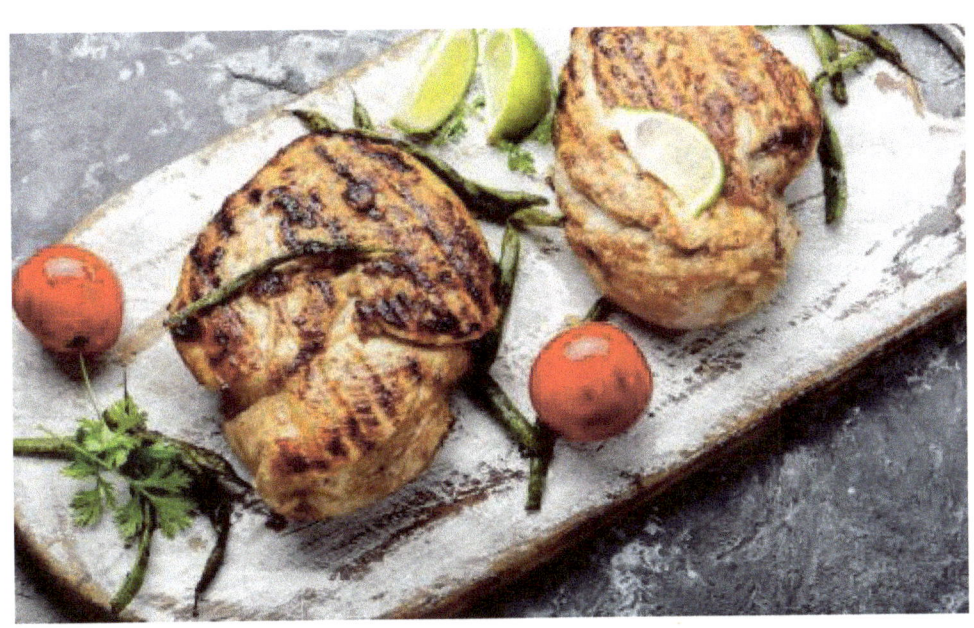

Chicken Fajitas

YIELD: SERVES 4

Festive fajitas make for a fast and satisfying meal. you can even use leftover chicken from another recipe, just warm it in a preheated 350°f oven for about 5 minutes.

Ingredients

2 organic chicken breasts

1 tsp organic cold-pressed olive oil

2 tsp chili powder

½ tsp cumin

½ tsp dried oregano

¼ tsp salt

¼ tsp freshly ground black pepper

2 cups grilled peppers and onions *(see next recipe)*

1 head butter or Boston bibb lettuce

2 limes, cut into wedges

Instructions

Rub the chicken with olive oil.

Season with chili powder, cumin, oregano, salt, and black pepper.

Heat a large skillet or grill over medium heat.

Cook the chicken for 8–10 minutes (or less for thinner cuts),
turning occasionally, until cooked through.

Transfer to a cutting board and let rest for 5 minutes. Slice thinly against th grain.

Separate the lettuce into leaves.

Place 2 slices of chicken and a spoonful of peppers and onions into each leaf.
Repeat with the remaining chicken and lettuce leaves.

Serve with lime wedges.

Buffalo Chicken Fingers

YIELD: 4 SERVINGS

This restaurant-inspired spin on Buffalo wings, minus the greasy skin and breading will have any finger-food fan clamoring for more. Broccoli fills out the meal, but these tasty chicken fingers can also be served over a leftover salad.

Ingredients

3 (6 oz) boneless, skinless chicken breasts, cut into strips

¼ tsp salt

¼ tsp freshly ground black pepper

1 Tbsp extra virgin cold-pressed olive oil

¼ cup gluten-free hot sauce

2 Tbsp tomato paste

4 Tbsp water

4 Tbsp unsalted ghee *(preferably grass–fed)*

4 cups broccoli florets or bok choy, chopped

Instructions

Sprinkle the chicken with salt and pepper.

Heat a large skillet over medium-high heat.

Add the olive oil, chicken, and broccoli. Cook for a few minutes, turning occasionally, until the chicken and broccoli begin to brown.

Reduce the heat to low. Stir in the hot sauce, tomato paste, and water. Mix well.

Add the ghee and stir until melted. Continue cooking until the sauce thickens and coats the chicken and broccoli.

Serve immediately.

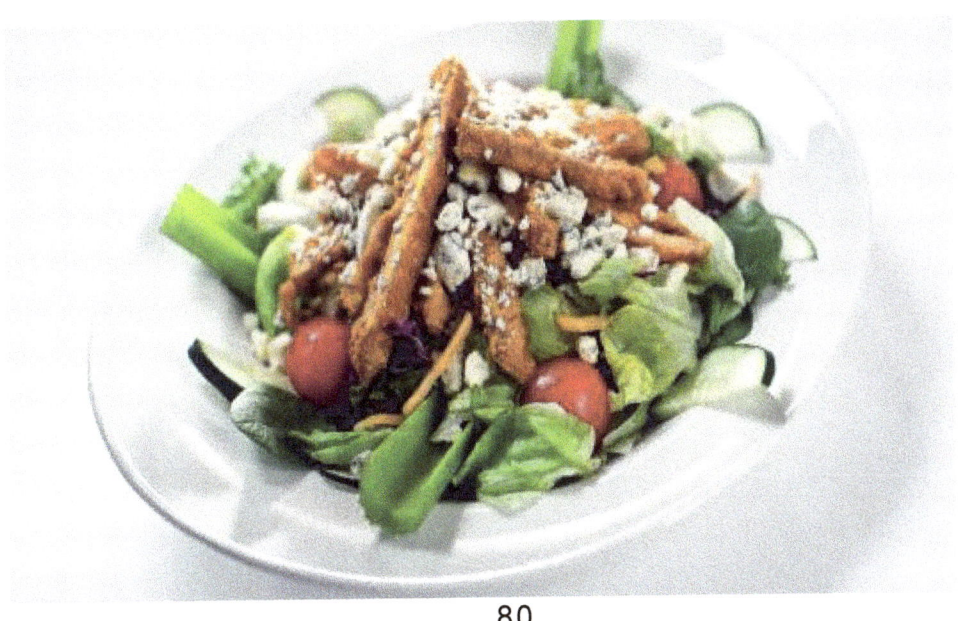

Chicken Salad Stuffed Peppers

YIELD: 4 SERVINGS

This healthier version of chicken salad makes a terrific lunch. The peppers not only add flavor and freshness but also bring a beautiful presentation to the plate!

Ingredients

For the Mayonnaise

1 large egg

1 Tbsp Dijon mustard

1 Tbsp lemon juice

¼ tsp fine sea salt or celery salt

1 cup very light olive oil *(the lighter, the better)*

For the Chicken Salad

½ cup homemade mayonnaise

1 ½ cups cooked chicken, diced

3 Tbsp red onion, finely diced

4 hard-boiled eggs, chopped

3 Tbsp diced pimento-stuffed green olives

½ tsp Dijon mustard *(or 1 tsp dry mustard powder)*

⅓ cup lemon juice

1 handful fresh dill, chopped

1 cucumber, peeled and cut into chunks

Artichoke hearts, chopped

4 bell peppers, hollowed out

Instructions

To Make the Mayonnaise

Add the egg, Dijon mustard, lemon juice, salt, and olive oil to a wide-mouth Mason jar, making sure the oil sits on top.

Place an immersion blender at the bottom of the jar and blend.

As the mayonnaise emulsifies, slowly tilt the blender to incorporate the remaining oil.

Store any unused portion in an airtight container in the refrigerator for up to two weeks.

To Make the Chicken Salad

Hollow the bell peppers by slicing off the tops, removing the veins, and tapping out the seeds.

In a mixing bowl, combine the mayonnaise, mustard, chicken, hard-boiled eggs, olives, red onion, cucumber, dill, and artichoke hearts. Mix well.

Spoon equal portions of the chicken salad into the 4 hollowed peppers.

Serve immediately.

Chicken Marsala (Balsamic Twist)

YIELD: 4 SERVINGS
(About 2 ½ Cups Per Serving)

Chicken Marsala gets its rich flavor from mushrooms and Marsala wine. This version is loaded with detoxifying mushrooms but swaps the wine for balsamic vinegar, giving it a tangy, flavorful twist.

Ingredients

4 skinless, boneless raw chicken cutlets
1 tsp dried oregano
¼ tsp salt
¼ tsp freshly ground black pepper
2 Tbsp extra virgin olive oil
2 cloves garlic, minced
2 Tbsp ghee *(preferably grass–fed)*
½ red or yellow onion, thinly sliced (about ½ cup)
1 small zucchini, thinly sliced
8 oz oyster mushrooms, sliced *(or more—mushrooms are always a great addition)*
1 Tbsp balsamic vinegar mixed with ⅓ cup water
¼ cup fresh basil, thinly sliced
Ground flaxseed, for sprinkling
Cooked barley, brown rice, black rice, or wild rice.

Instructions

Heat olive oil in a large skillet over medium-high heat.
Sprinkle the chicken with oregano, salt, and pepper.
Add the chicken and garlic to the skillet. Cook for 2–3 minutes, turning once, until lightly browned.
Add the ghee, onion, zucchini, and mushrooms. Cook for another 2–3 minutes, until the vegetables soften. Sprinkle with ground flaxseed.
Stir well, then add the balsamic vinegar–water mixture.
Cook for 1 more minute, until the sauce thickens slightly. Sprinkle with fresh basil.
Serve immediately over your choice of barley, wild rice, brown rice, or black rice.
For extra flavor, cook the grains in organic chicken broth instead of water.

Grilled Chicken Thighs in Tomato Sauce

A rich, flavorful tomato sauce over tender chicken thighs that will make you feel good all over!

Ingredients

2 ripe tomatoes, halved
1 large red bell pepper, seeded and quartered
½ cup sun-dried tomato strips in oil, well drained
Small handful of fresh basil leaves
1 large clove of garlic, crushed
1 tsp dried oregano *(or 1 Tbsp fresh)*
¼ tsp salt
¼ tsp freshly ground black pepper
3 Tbsp extra virgin olive oil (EVOO)
6-8 chicken thighs, bone-in

Instructions

Preheat the grill to high.
In a food processor, combine the tomatoes, bell pepper, sun-dried tomatoes, basil, garlic, oregano, salt, and pepper.
Drizzle the olive oil over the mixture.
Pulse a few times to break up large pieces, then process steadily, scraping down the sides as needed, until the mixture forms a mostly smooth sauce.
If the sauce is too thick, add more oil, one teaspoon at a time, until you reach the desired consistency.
Taste and adjust seasoning if necessary. Set aside.
Season the chicken thighs lightly with salt and pepper.
Place the chicken on the hottest part of the grill and cook undisturbed for 4-5 minutes, until opaque.
Flip and cook another 4-5 minutes, until just cooked through.
Allow the chicken to rest, covered, for at least 5 minutes.
Top with sauce to taste and serve.

Serving Suggestions

This dish is delicious over zucchini noodles or cabbage. Crockpot Variation: Prepare the tomato sauce as directed. Place the sauce in the crockpot, then add the seasoned chicken. Cook for 6-8 hours (start on high until bubbly, then reduce to medium). Add cabbage or zucchini during the last 2 hours of cooking, making sure to season well. For extra heat, add red pepper flakes.

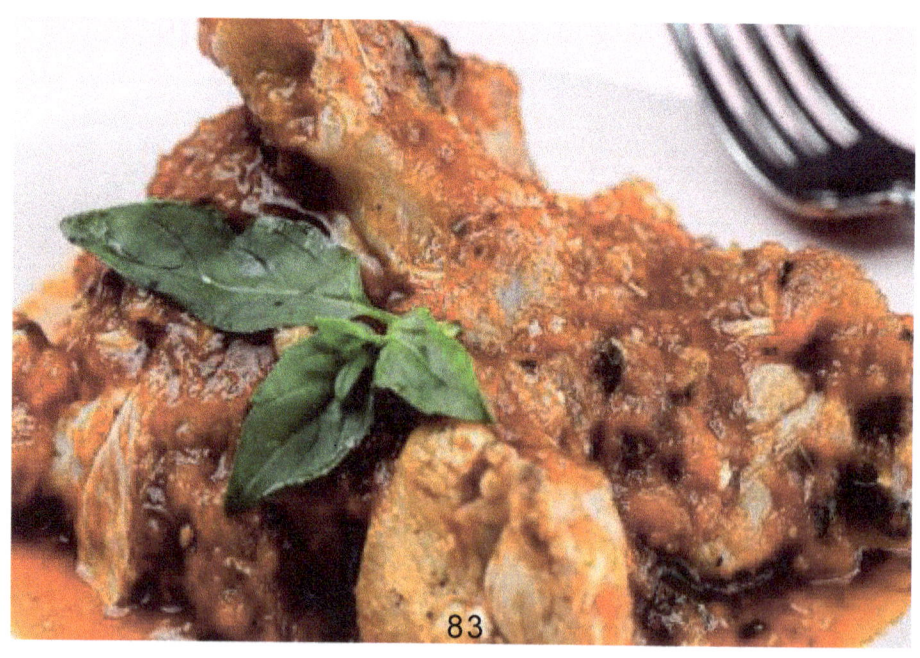

Chicken Fried Rice

YIELD: 4 SERVINGS
(About 2 ½ Cups Per Serving)

This version of fried rice will have you craving homemade instead of takeout. Knowing exactly what's in your food and how it's prepared offers peace of mind. Short on time? Choosing organic frozen vegetables is always a win since they retain their nutritional value. You can also double up on the rice and freeze.

Ingredients

½ lb raw, unbreaded chicken tenders
1 tsp Chinese Five Spice
Organic garlic powder, to taste
Organic olive oil spray
1 egg, scrambled with 1 egg white
8 cups organic jasmine rice, cooked
1 cup fresh organic green beans, chopped
½ cup organic baby peas
1 cup shredded carrots
Bragg's Liquid Aminos spray *(non–soy alternative)*
Optional: 8 oz frozen mixed vegetables (e.g., green beans, peas, carrots)

Instructions

- Cut the chicken tenders into ½-inch slices and transfer to a plate.
- Sprinkle with Chinese Five Spice and garlic powder.
- Heat a large skillet over medium-high heat and spray with olive oil (or coconut oil).
- Add the chicken and cook for 4–5 minutes, stirring often, until no longer pink and cooked through.
- Add the egg and egg white mixture, cooking for 1 minute more while stirring continuously until scrambled and fully cooked.
- Add the cooked rice and vegetables along with ¼ cup of water.
- Reduce the heat to low and cook for 2 more minutes, until the vegetables are heated through.
- Spray with Bragg's Liquid Aminos to taste, toss well, and serve immediately.

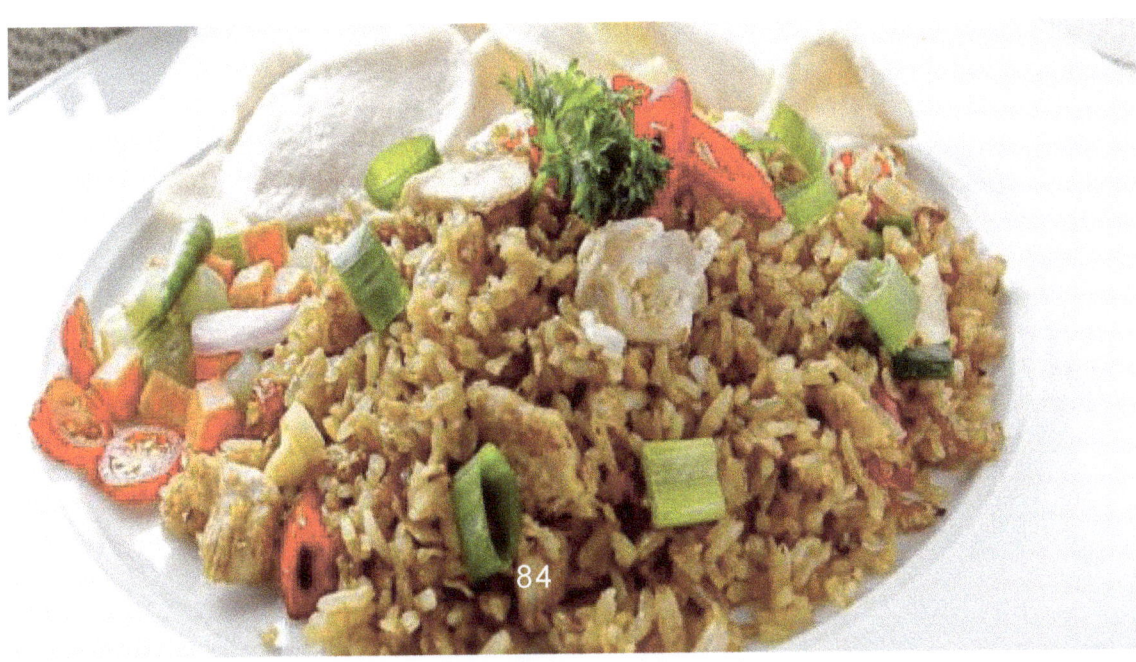

Chicken Cacciatore

"Cacciatore" means hunter-style. Traditionally, hunters made this dish with mushrooms they found in the forest. This quick version takes under 20 minutes to prepare and works well with any type of mushrooms, whether store-bought or freshly foraged.

Ingredients

¾ lb chicken breasts (about 4 breasts)

1 tsp oregano

1 tsp thyme

1 tsp basil

1 tsp rosemary, chopped (fresh or dried)

¼ tsp freshly ground black pepper

¼ tsp salt

3 Tbsp ghee

1 lb mushrooms, thinly sliced (or more, to taste)

½ red bell pepper, thinly sliced

¼ cup onion, thinly sliced

1 tsp garlic powder

4 cups baby spinach or chopped kale

1 Tbsp fresh lemon juice

2 cloves garlic, chopped

Instructions

Preheat oven or toaster oven to 400°F (200°C).

Line a baking sheet with aluminum foil.

Season the chicken with oregano, rosemary, black pepper, salt, and garlic powder.

Place the chicken skin-side up on the prepared baking sheet.

Bake for 30-35 minutes, or until the chicken is no longer pink at the bone.

While the chicken cooks, prepare the sauce:

Warm the ghee in a large skillet over medium heat.

Add mushrooms, bell pepper, onion, chopped garlic, thyme, and basil.

Cook for 3-4 minutes, stirring until the mushrooms begin to soften and the onions brown.

Turn off the heat, add the lemon juice, and toss well.

To serve: Place 2 cups of spinach or kale on each plate. Top with the chicken and spoon the mushroom sauce over. Serve immediately.

Crockpot Variation

For an easy slow-cooked version:

Brown the chicken first, then place it in the crockpot with all the ingredients. Add 1 each of yellow, green, and red bell peppers, thinly sliced. Cook on low for about 6 hours, until the chicken falls apart. Serve over mashed cauliflower for a hearty, comforting meal.

Turkey Breast Slowly Cooked

YIELD: 6 SERVINGS
(2 Slices Per Serving)

No one likes dry meat, and with this recipe, you'll impress yourself. Set your slow cooker to low and let it do the work. Since turkey breasts (or pork loins) are usually 2½–3 pounds, you'll also have delicious leftovers for lunch.

Ingredients

2 tbsp nutmeg

2 tbsp rosemary (fresh or dried, chopped)

4 cloves garlic, thinly sliced

1 tbsp onion powder

1 cup vegetable broth
Salt and pepper, to taste

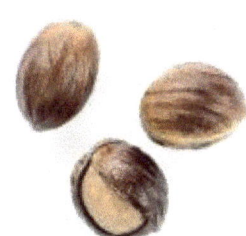

Instructions

● Place the vegetable broth in the bottom of the slow cooker.

● Season the turkey breast by sprinkling nutmeg, rosemary, onion powder, garlic, salt, and pepper on top.

● Cover and set the slow cooker to **low**. Cook for 3–3½ hours, until the turkey is cooked through but still very slightly pink in the center.

● Transfer the roast to a cutting board and let it rest for 5 minutes before slicing.

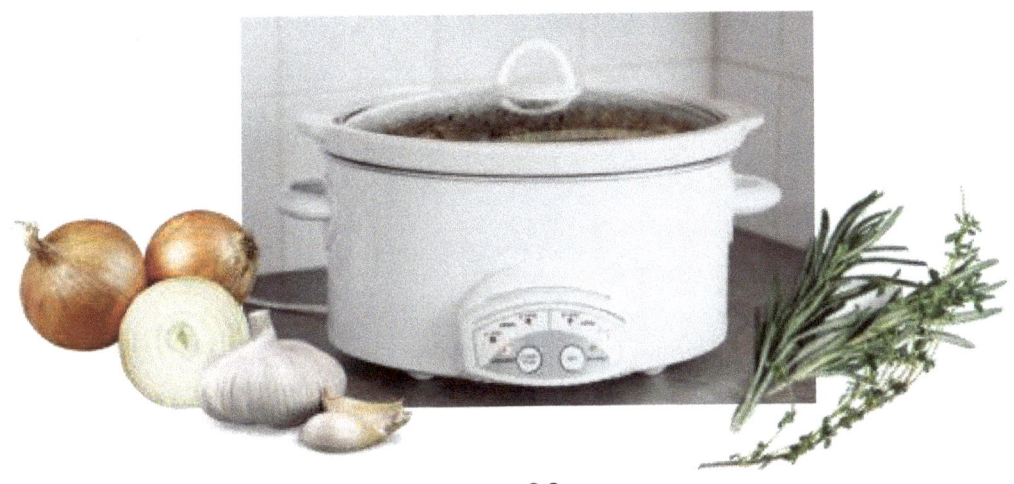

Turkey Chili

YIELD: 3 SERVINGS

Fresh cilantro and lime give this chili a burst of flavor. It keeps well in the refrigerator for up to five days and can also be frozen in two-cup portions. Leftovers make an easy, no-hassle lunch.

Ingredients

2 tbsp olive oil (or coconut oil)

1 lb ground turkey

½ cup fresh cilantro, chopped (dried can also be used)

½ yellow or red onion, finely chopped

3 garlic cloves, minced

2 tbsp chili powder (mild or hot)

2 tsp ground cumin

1 tsp oregano (or 1 tbsp fresh)

6 tbsp tomato paste (or fresh tomatoes)

32 oz low-sodium, gluten-free chicken broth

1 (15 oz) can diced tomatoes (or fresh)

1 small zucchini, sliced or grated (grating helps thicken the chili)

1 cup kale, stemmed and chopped (or torn into bite-sized pieces)

¼ cup fresh lime juice (about 2 limes, adjust to taste)

1 large or 2 small cans of kidney beans

Instructions

Heat oil in a stockpot over medium heat. Brown ground turkey for 1-2 minutes, then add cilantro, onion, and garlic; cook 2-3 minutes, breaking up the meat. Stir in chili powder, cumin, oregano, and tomato paste; cook 1 minute. Add broth, tomatoes, zucchini, kale, and beans; simmer 20-30 minutes until meat is cooked and veggies are tender. Finish with lime juice and serve.

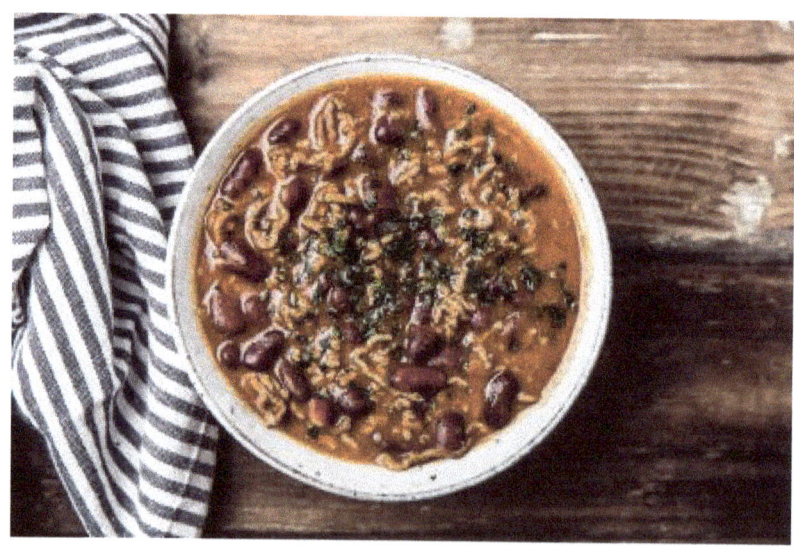

Meatloaf

YIELD: 4 SERVINGS
(2 Slices Per Person)

This classically American dish is usually made with bread, but this version uses grated zucchini to keep it moist, lower the calories, and add incredible flavor. No one will even know it's in there!

Ingredients

Organic olive oil spray (or coconut oil spray)
1 small yellow or red onion, finely chopped
3 garlic cloves, minced
1 cup zucchini, grated (about 1 small zucchini)
1 lb ground turkey
1 egg
1 tsp chili powder (mild or hot)
½ tsp dried oregano (or 1 tsp fresh)
¼ tsp freshly ground black pepper
½ tsp celery salt
1 tbsp tomato paste mixed with 1 tsp olive oil
⅓ cup ground flaxseed (optional, helps bind the loaf)
1 tsp ground cumin
1 tsp extra virgin cold-pressed olive oil

Instructions

Preheat the oven to 400°F (200°C).

Heat a large skillet over medium-high heat and spray with olive oil or coconut oil spray.

Add the onion, garlic, chili powder, oregano, black pepper, celery salt, and cumin. Cook for 3–4 minutes, stirring often, until the vegetables soften and begin to brown.

Transfer the mixture to a large bowl and let cool slightly, about 5 minutes.

Add the grated zucchini and toss to combine.

Add the ground turkey, egg, and flaxseed (if using). Mix well and shape into a loaf.

Transfer to a baking dish and spread the tomato paste–olive oil mixture evenly on top.

Bake for 45-50 minutes, until the meatloaf is firm at the edges and cooked through. Let rest for 5–10 minutes before slicing and serving.

Roasted Turkey (In a Crock Pot)

A tender roast can be as easy as switching on your slow cooker and adding flavorful spices and fill your home with a wonderful aroma.

Ingredients

1 organic turkey breast

1 yellow or red onion, coarsely chopped

3 celery stalks, sliced

1 (14 oz) can diced tomatoes

3 tbsp lemon juice

2 tbsp tomato paste

1 tbsp Dijon mustard

4 garlic cloves, crushed and chopped

2 carrots, diced

8 oz mushrooms, sliced

½ tsp salt

½ tsp freshly ground black pepper

1 tsp fresh rosemary, chopped

1 cup organic turkey broth

¼ tsp cumin

¼ tsp turmeric

1 tsp chili powder, hot (optional)

Alternative Seasoning Mix (instead of cumin, turmeric, and chili powder):

1 tsp thyme

1 tsp basil

1 tsp. parsley

¼ tsp celery salt

1 bulb fennel, sliced

1 bay leaf

Instructions

●   Place the turkey breast in the slow cooker (no added water needed).

●   Add all remaining ingredients.

●   Use a rubber spatula to spread and coat the turkey breast with the seasonings and vegetables.

●   Cover and cook on low for 6–8 hours, or until the turkey is cooked through and tender.

●   Slice and serve with a salad or vegetable side dish.

Tip:

Leftovers make an excellent base for turkey soup, see the soups section for recipe ideas.

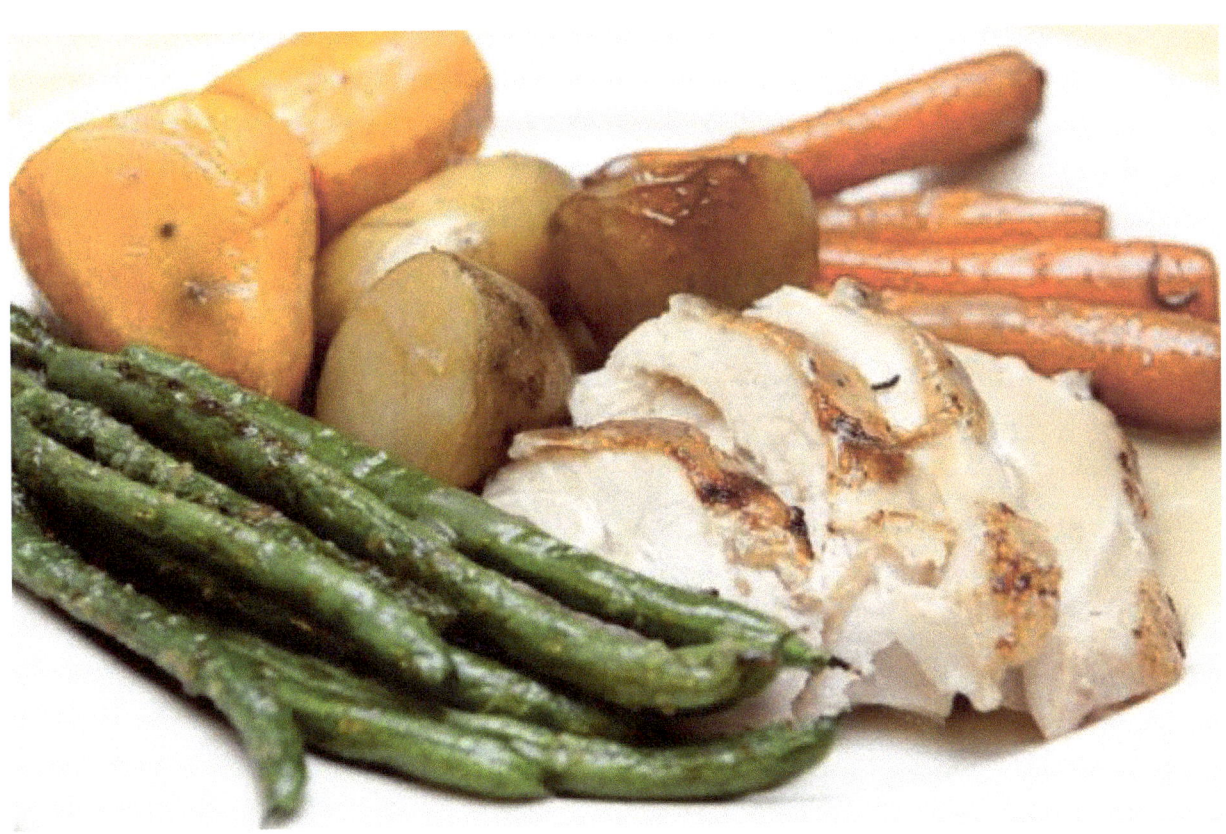

Pasta Bolognese

Bolognese is a rich, savory meat sauce that's surprisingly quick to make. Chop the vegetables in advance, or use a food processor to cut prep time in half. Finish with fresh basil leaves for extra flavor.

Ingredients

8 oz gluten-free pasta (such as red lentil pasta)

1 tsp olive oil

1 lb lean ground turkey (90%) or organic chicken

4 carrots, peeled and chopped

3 celery stalks, peeled and chopped

1 medium onion, chopped

12 oz mushrooms, sliced or diced

1 (6 oz) can tomato paste

1 (28 oz) can diced tomatoes

½ cup grated Parmesan

Instructions

Heat a large stockpot over medium-high heat. Add the olive oil, then the ground turkey or chicken. Cook for 2–3 minutes, stirring until the meat begins to brown.

Reduce the heat to medium. Add the carrots, celery, mushrooms, and onion. Cook for about 5 minutes, stirring often, until the vegetables are soft.

Stir in the tomato paste and cook for 1 minute, until fragrant.

Add the diced tomatoes along with 1 cup of water. Stir well.

Bring to a simmer over medium-low heat. Cook for 20–25 minutes, until the sauce is thick and hearty.

While the sauce is simmering, cook the pasta according to package directions.

Tip: For gluten-free pasta, cook 1–2 minutes less than directed to prevent sogginess.

Drain well. Toss the pasta with the sauce and top with grated Parmesan.

Chef's Notes: Avoid cooking gluten-free pasta ahead of time, as it can turn mushy. Recommended brands with great texture: *Pasta Joy Rice Pasta, Bonanaturae Potato Pasta, and Boles Corn Pasta.*

For a lighter option, serve the sauce over steamed cabbage with shredded carrots.

Fish

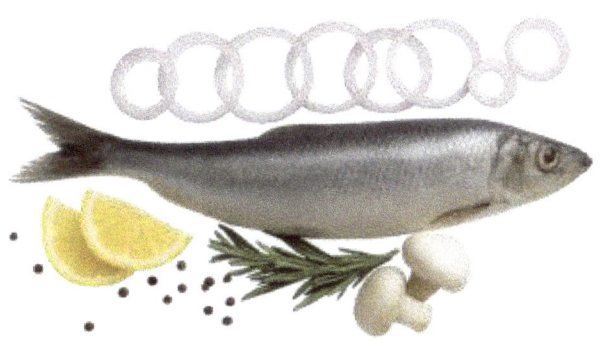

Fish rich in omega-3 fatty acids may play an important role in lowering the risk of breast cancer recurrence and improving survival in those who have had breast cancer. Omega-3s are also powerful anti-inflammatory compounds, and since chronic inflammation can contribute to cancer progression, they offer an additional layer of protection. Research published in the *Journal of Nutrition* found that women with higher omega-3 intake from fish had a 25% lower risk of breast cancer. Other studies show that the omega-3 fatty acids EPA and DHA found primarily in fatty fish can slow the growth and progression of breast tumors.

Fatty fish such as salmon, sardines, and mackerel are especially beneficial. They provide not only omega-3s, but also selenium and antioxidants like astaxanthin, which together help defend the body against cancer and support overall health. Regularly including these fish in your diet may significantly lower your risk of breast cancer while promoting long-term wellness.

Arctic Char With Fresh Cilantro Pesto

YIELD: 4 SERVINGS

Arctic char has a delicate, slightly sweet flavor that pairs beautifully with the rich, nutty taste of pistachios and the bright freshness of cilantro. This dish is not only full of flavor but also packed with heart-healthy Omega-3s.

Ingredients

1 ½ cups fresh cilantro, packed

Juice of 1 small lime

⅓ cup pistachios, shelled

Olive oil, for drizzling

4 Arctic char fillets

Montreal steak seasoning, to taste

Instructions

Preheat the grill to medium heat.

In a food processor, combine cilantro, lime juice, and pistachios. Process until finely chopped, scraping down the sides as needed. With the motor running, drizzle in olive oil until the mixture reaches a smooth, pesto-like consistency.

Lightly season the fish with Montreal steak seasoning.

Grill the fillets for 6-8 minutes per side (depending on thickness), until the fish is opaque and flakes easily with a fork.

Spread a thick layer of pistachio-cilantro pesto over the fish. Serve immediately, with extra pesto on the side.

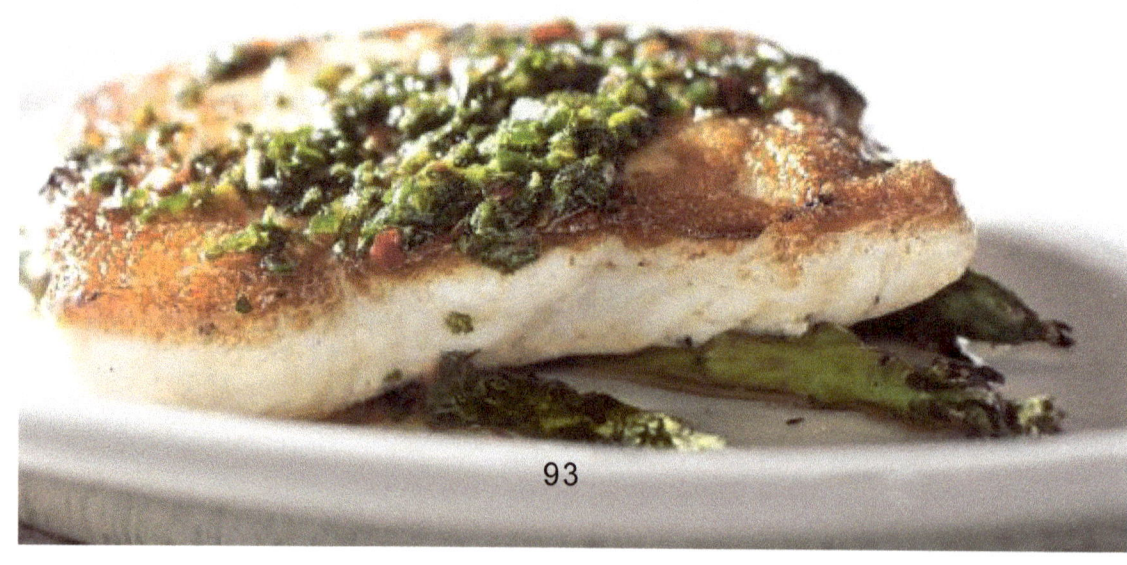

Citrus Mackerel with Garlicky Collard Greens

A bold, flavorful dish that balances the richness of mackerel with the bright, tangy taste of citrus and the earthy depth of garlicky greens. Packed with Omega-3s, fiber, and antioxidants, this meal is as nourishing as it is delicious.

Ingredients

For the Mackerel

Fresh organic mackerel fillets

1 Tbsp. olive oil *or* walnut oil

1 clove garlic, minced

½ tsp. black pepper

½ tsp. smoked paprika

½ tsp. celery salt

½ tsp. onion powder

Juice & zest of 1 lemon or lime (or use ½ an orange for a sweeter twist)

1 Tbsp. fresh parsley or cilantro, chopped (optional)

For the Garlicky Collard Greens

1 bunch collard greens, chopped

1 Tbsp. olive oil

2-3 cloves garlic, minced

½ tsp. black pepper

Juice of ½ lemon, lime or orange juice

¼ tsp. crushed red pepper flakes (optional, for heat)

Instructions

Cook the Mackerel

Heat olive oil in a skillet over medium heat.

Rub the mackerel fillets with garlic, black pepper, paprika, celery salt, onion powder, and citrus zest.

Place the fillets skin-side down in the pan and cook for 3-4 minutes. Flip and cook for another 3 minutes, or until the fish is opaque and flakes easily.

Finish with a squeeze of fresh citrus juice and garnish with parsley or cilantro.

Saute the Collard Greens

While the fish is cooking, heat olive oil in another skillet over medium heat.

Add garlic and sauté for 30 seconds, until fragrant.

Add the chopped collard greens and stir well. Cook for 5-7 minutes, until wilted and tender.

Season with black pepper, crushed red pepper, and a squeeze of lemon, lime, or orange juice.

Tip:

Swap collard greens for kale, Swiss chard, or spinach if preferred.

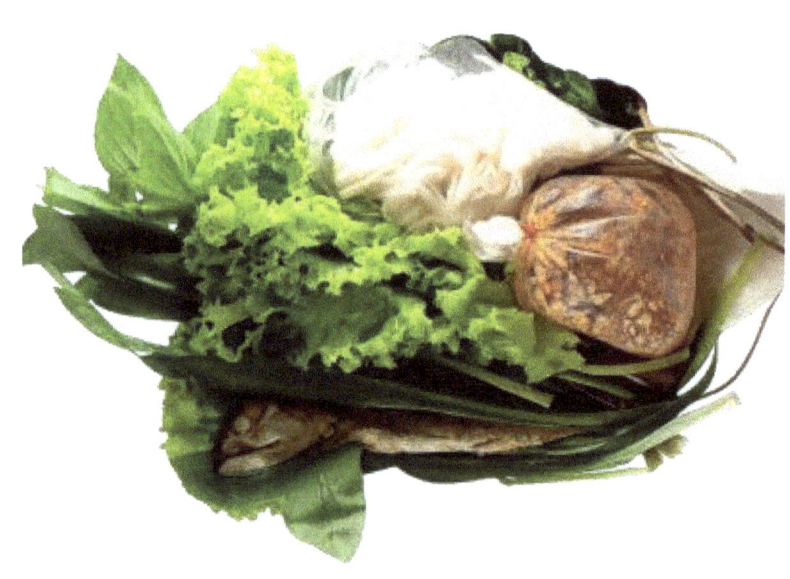

Lake Trout with Onion-Herb Cauliflower Mash Roasted Brussels Sprouts & Carrots

A wholesome, flavorful meal that balances tender lake trout with creamy cauliflower mash and caramelized roasted vegetables. Rich in protein, fiber, and antioxidants. It's as nourishing as it is delicious.

Ingredients

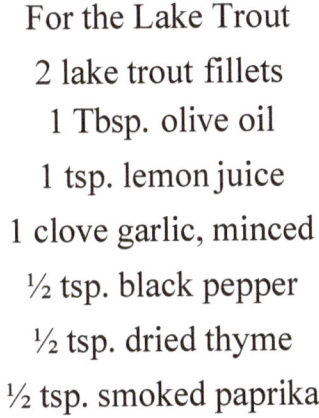

For the Lake Trout

2 lake trout fillets

1 Tbsp. olive oil

1 tsp. lemon juice

1 clove garlic, minced

½ tsp. black pepper

½ tsp. dried thyme

½ tsp. smoked paprika

For the Onion-Herb Cauliflower Mash

1 medium head cauliflower, chopped

1 small onion, finely diced

1 Tbsp. olive oil or unsalted butter

½ tsp. garlic powder

½ tsp. dried parsley *or* fresh

½ tsp. black pepper

For the Roasted Brussels Sprouts

1 cup Brussels Sprouts,

1 cup carrots, sliced

1 Tbsp. olive oil

½ tsp. black pepper

½ tsp fresh or dried rosemary

Instructions

Prepare the Onion-Herb Cauliflower Mash

Steam or boil the cauliflower until soft, about 10 minutes.

In a pan, sauté the onion in olive oil until golden.

Blend the cauliflower with sautéed onion, garlic powder, parsley, black pepper, and a drizzle of olive oil until smooth. Set aside.

Roast the Brussels Sprouts & Carrots

Preheat oven to 400°F (200°C).

Toss Brussels Sprouts and carrots with olive oil, black pepper, and rosemary.

Spread on a baking sheet and roast for 20-25 minutes, flipping halfway through.

Cook the Lake Trout

Heat olive oil in a skillet over medium heat.

Rub trout fillets with lemon juice, garlic, black pepper, thyme, and paprika.

Place fillets skin-side down and cook for 3-4 minutes. Flip and cook for another 3 minutes, or until the fish flakes easily with a fork.

Assemble

Plate the trout alongside the cauliflower mash and roasted vegetables.

Serve immediately and enjoy!

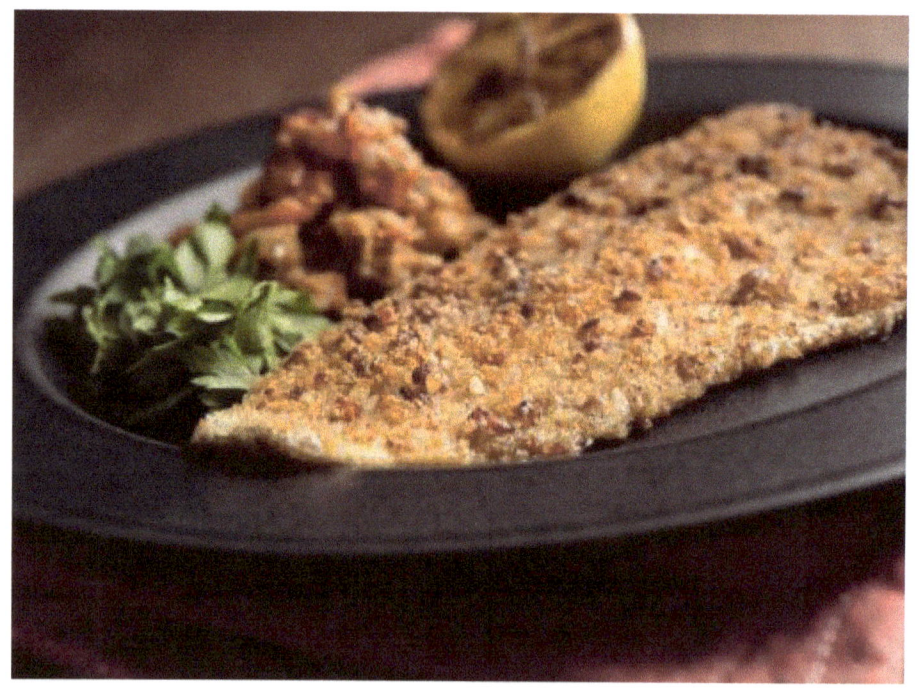

Spicy Herring with Roasted Veggies

A bold and zesty dish that pairs the rich flavor of herring with warm spices and a refreshing citrus finish. Perfect served with roasted vegetables for a wholesome, nutrient-packed meal.

Ingredients

Fresh or canned herring fillets

1 Tbsp. olive oil

1 clove garlic, minced

½ tsp. ground cumin

½ tsp. ground coriander

½ tsp. ground turmeric

½ tsp. chili flakes (optional, for extra heat)

Zest and juice of 1 orange

1 Tbsp. chopped fresh cilantro or parsley

Instructions

In a small bowl, combine cumin, coriander, turmeric, and chili flakes.

Rub the herring fillets with minced garlic, the spice blend, and orange zest.

Heat olive oil in a skillet over medium heat.

Place the fillets skin-side down and cook for 3-4 minutes. Flip and cook for another 3 minutes, or until fish is opaque and flakes easily.

Squeeze fresh orange juice over the fillets and garnish with chopped cilantro or parsley.

Serve hot with roasted vegetables on the side.

Tips & Variations

For extra flavor, marinate the herring in the spice mix and orange juice for 20 minutes before cooking.

Pair with roasted carrots, zucchini, or bell peppers for a colorful plate.

If using canned herring, reduce cooking time to just warming through in the skillet.

Herb Roasted Vegetables

A colorful, flavorful mix of roasted vegetables seasoned with herbs and finished with a bright citrus drizzle. Perfect as a side dish for chicken, fish, or plant-based mains.

Ingredients

1 cup carrots, sliced

1 cup Brussels sprouts, halved

1 zucchini, cut into large pieces

1 small red onion, sliced

1 Tbsp. olive oil (or walnut oil)

½ tsp. dried rosemary

½ tsp. dried thyme

½ tsp. black pepper

Salt to taste

Juice of ½ lemon or lime

Instructions

Preheat oven to 400°F (200°C).

Toss the carrots, Brussels sprouts, zucchini, and red onion with olive oil, rosemary, and thyme. Season with salt and black pepper. Spread the vegetables in a single layer on a baking sheet.

Roast for 20-25 minutes, flipping halfway through, until tender and lightly browned.

Drizzle with lemon or lime juice before serving.

Salmon Dinner with Cauliflower Mash

So good, and so good for you!
This creamy cauliflower mash pairs perfectly with tender, seared salmon for a wholesome, satisfying meal.

Ingredients
For the Cauliflower Mash
1 head of cauliflower, cut into florets
2 Tbsp. unsalted butter (preferably grass-fed)
¼ cup scallions, chopped
1 tsp. salt (divided)
1 tsp. freshly ground black pepper (divided)
For the Salmon
4 salmon fillets or steaks
1 tsp. olive oil

Instructions
Cauliflower Mash (Stovetop Method)

Place 1 inch of water in a large stockpot and bring to a boil.

Add the cauliflower, cover, and cook for 3-4 minutes, until tender and most of the water has evaporated.

Reduce the heat to medium, remove the lid, and add butter, scallions, and half the salt and pepper.

Cover again and cook for 1 minute more, until any residual water has cooked off.

Remove from heat and mash with a mixer until smooth.
Cauliflower Mash (Microwave Method - Alternative)
Cut cauliflower into very small florets and place in a microwave-safe bowl.

Cover with a very damp paper towel.

Microwave for 7-12 minutes, until very soft.

Transfer to a food processor and blend with butter, scallions, and half the salt and pepper until smooth.

Salmon

Sprinkle salmon with the remaining salt and pepper.
Heat a medium skillet over high heat. Add olive oil and the salmon. Lower the heat to medium and cook 3-4 minutes without turning. Flip and cook another 3-4 minutes to sear the other side. Continue cooking an additional 8-10 minutes, turning occasionally, until the salmon is cooked to your desired doneness. Remove from heat, let rest for 5 minutes, and serve with cauliflower mash.

Pistachio Crusted Salmon

This dish is tasty, moist, and oh-so good for you. Serve with roasted vegetables and a fresh salad for a wholesome, balanced meal.

Ingredients

4 (4-oz.) salmon fillets, skin on

2–4 Tbsp. mustard, mixed with 20 drops of toffee stevia

1 clove garlic, finely chopped

4 Tbsp. chopped pistachios (or substitute walnuts, almonds, or macadamias)

¼ cup scallions, thinly sliced

Everything Bagel seasoning, to taste

Instructions

Preheat the oven to 400°F (200°C).

Place the salmon, skin-side down, in a baking dish.

In a small bowl, mix the mustard, stevia, and garlic.

Spread the mustard mixture over each fillet.

Sprinkle with Everything Bagel seasoning, then top each fillet with 1 Tbsp. of chopped nuts.

Bake for 10–12 minutes, until the salmon is pink in the center but not translucent. For well-done salmon, cook an additional 2 minutes.

Remove from the oven, top with scallions, and let rest lightly covered for 5 minutes before serving.

Chefs Notes

You can also bake this salmon in a toaster oven.

Mix different nuts for a unique flavor twist.

Serve with a side of vegetables, a crisp salad, or barley with caramelized onions for a complete meal.

Salmon Burger

YIELD: 4 SERVINGS

These healthy burgers require very little prep time and are loaded with Omega-3s. Pair them with a side of vegetables for a heart- and brain-healthy meal.

Ingredients

1 egg

2 (7.5 oz.) cans wild salmon (*fresh is even better!*)

⅓ cup almond flour

1 Tbsp. lemon zest

1 Tbsp. fresh dill, finely chopped

1 Tbsp. capers, rinsed and drained (optional)

1 tsp. smoked paprika

1 tsp. Dijon mustard or Dijonnaise

¼ cup onion, finely chopped

Olive oil, to lightly coat the pan

1 lemon, quartered

1 ripe avocado, sliced

1 tomato, sliced

Arugula

Instructions
For Canned Salmon

- In a medium bowl, lightly beat the egg.
- Add the salmon, almond flour, lemon zest, dill, capers, mustard, paprika, and onion. Mix well until thoroughly combined.
- Shape firmly into four patties.
- Lightly coat a large skillet with olive oil and place it over medium heat.
- Cook 4-5 minutes per side, until lightly browned and cooked through.
- If desired, squeeze fresh lemon juice over the patties.
- Serve on a bed of arugula, topped with sliced tomato and avocado.

For Fresh Salmon (Alternative Method)

- Preheat oven to 350°F (175°C). Line a baking sheet with parchment paper.
- Place wild-caught salmon fillets on the sheet and season with Montreal steak seasoning.
- Bake until the salmon flakes easily with a fork.
- Flake the cooked salmon into a medium bowl and follow the mixing and patty-shaping directions above.

Dijon Salmon Steaks

YIELD: 4 SERVINGS

Salmon is an excellent source of Omega-3s, which, when consumed regularly, can support cardiovascular, joint, brain, and even eye health. For the best quality, purchase wild salmon whenever possible, as it typically contains fewer contaminants.

Ingredients

4 (6 oz.) salmon steaks

1 lemon, halved

Salt and freshly ground black pepper, to taste

2 Tbsp. Dijon mustard

4 tsp. fresh dill, minced

Instructions

Preheat the broiler. Lightly coat a broiler rack with high-heat cooking spray and set aside.

Squeeze the lemon halves evenly over the salmon to coat with juice. Let it rest for 5 minutes.

Season the salmon steaks with salt and pepper, then arrange them on the prepared broiler rack.

Broil for about 4 minutes. Remove from the broiler pan, flip the steaks, and spread equal amounts of Dijon mustard over the tops.

Return to the broiler and cook for another 3-4 minutes, or until the salmon is just opaque and flakes easily with a fork.

Transfer the steaks to a serving platter and sprinkle with fresh dill before serving.

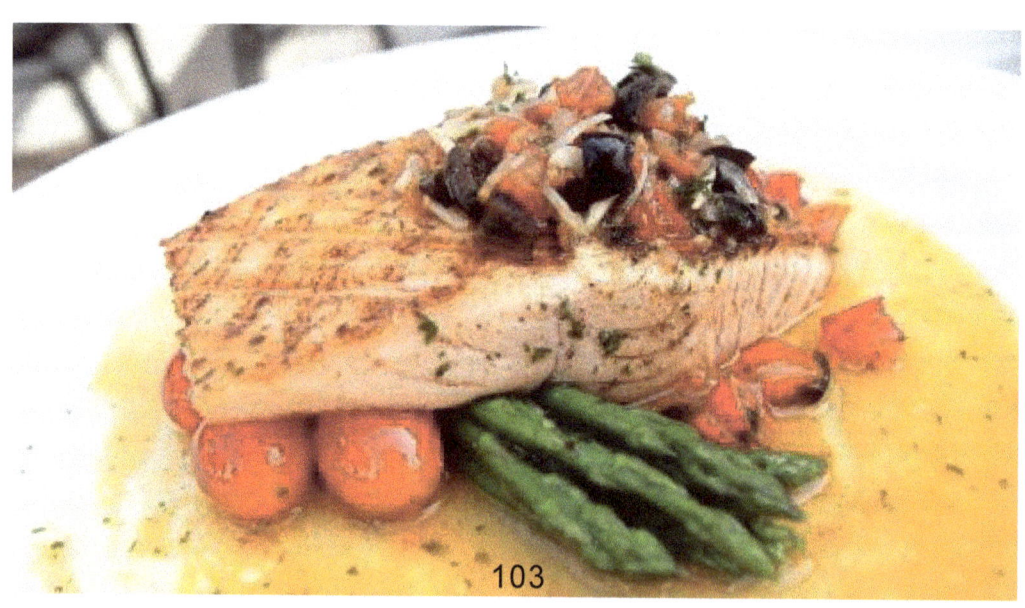

Coconut Salmon (Slow Cooker)

If cooking feels daunting, this easy slow cooker recipe is perfect. The slow cooker ensures the salmon stays tender and moist while infusing it with a rich, garlicky coconut sauce. A touch of chili adds gentle heat, but you can omit it if you prefer a milder flavor.

Ingredients

½ cup unsweetened coconut milk

2 scallions, thinly sliced

4 cloves garlic, minced

2 Tbsp. cold-pressed extra-virgin coconut oil

½ tsp. salt

¼ tsp. crushed red chili flakes (optional)

4 (4 oz.) salmon fillets, skin removed

1 Tbsp. parsley, minced

4 cups baby spinach

Instructions

Place the coconut milk, scallions, garlic, coconut oil, salt, and chili flakes (if using) in the slow cooker.

Stir well to combine.

Add the salmon fillets and turn gently to coat in the coconut mixture.

Set the slow cooker to low and cook for 2 hours, until the salmon is cooked through but still tender.

During the last 10 minutes of cooking, add the parsley and spinach on top of the salmon.

Garnish with freshly grated, unsweetened coconut.

Serve immediately.

Serving Suggestion

This dish is delicious served with black rice cooked in coconut milk or coconut water, so creamy and satisfying.

Breakfast,
Lunch Or Dinner

Breakfast is crucial for breast cancer patients because it provides the energy and nutrients needed to combat treatment side effects, helps maintain a healthy weight, and may even reduce cancer risk by supporting circadian rhythm regulation. Starting the day with a balanced meal also sets the tone for healthier eating patterns throughout the day and prevents excessive snacking or overeating later on.

Your body continues to burn energy while you sleep, and when you wake up, it needs replenishment. Breakfast provides the perfect opportunity to consume nutrient-rich foods that fuel your body with essential vitamins, minerals, and antioxidants, all of which support healing, immune function, and energy for recovery. Research shows that skipping breakfast can disrupt circadian rhythms, which may increase cancer risk. A recent study published in *Cancer Causes & Control* reported that people who regularly skipped breakfast had a higher incidence of cancer, greater cancer-related mortality, and an even higher risk of all-cause mortality. Clearly, breakfast is more than just a meal; it's an investment in your health and longevity. If breakfast feels unappealing, think about ways to expand your choices. The first meal of the day doesn't have to be limited to cereal, eggs, or toast. Around the world, many cultures start the day with hearty foods like soups, fish, or vegetables. Smoothies are another excellent option, offering hydration along with concentrated nutrients that help fight cancer and restore strength.

Most importantly, eat what tastes good to you within the boundaries of cancer-fighting foods (like those in this cookbook!). Consistency matters more than perfection. Fueling your body every morning is a simple yet powerful step toward healing and resilience.

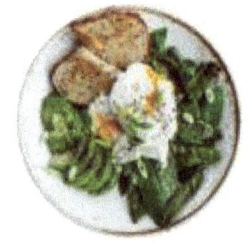 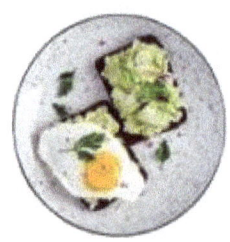 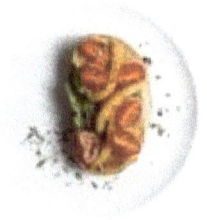 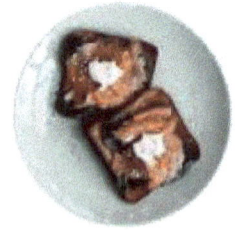

Huevos Rancheros

YIELD: 4 SERVINGS
Gluten-Free

Huevos Rancheros are the Mexican version of a classic "eggs and sausage" breakfast. This lighter version skips the sausage (chorizo) but still delivers the bold Latin flavors everyone loves. Thanks to salsa, cilantro, beans, and warm tortillas.

Ingredients

4 Corn tortillas
4 Eggs
1 Tbsp. olive oil (or coconut oil)
1 (14 oz.) can refried beans, butter beans,
or kidney beans
1 cup of organic brown rice, cooked
½ cup feta cheese, crumbled
¼ cup fresh cilantro leaves
½ cup salsa (mild, medium, or hot, to taste)

Instructions

Heat olive oil in a large skillet over medium heat.
Crack the eggs gently into the skillet and cook for 3-4 minutes for sunny-side-up eggs (or longer if you prefer firmer yolks). Sprinkle with feta cheese and set aside.
In a separate skillet, warm the beans and rice together. Stir in the cilantro.
Warm the tortillas in a toaster oven or a preheated oven at 350°F for about 5 minutes.

To Assemble

Place one tortilla on each plate. Top with an egg, a spoonful of beans and rice, a sprinkle of feta, and a generous spoonful of salsa. Serve immediately.

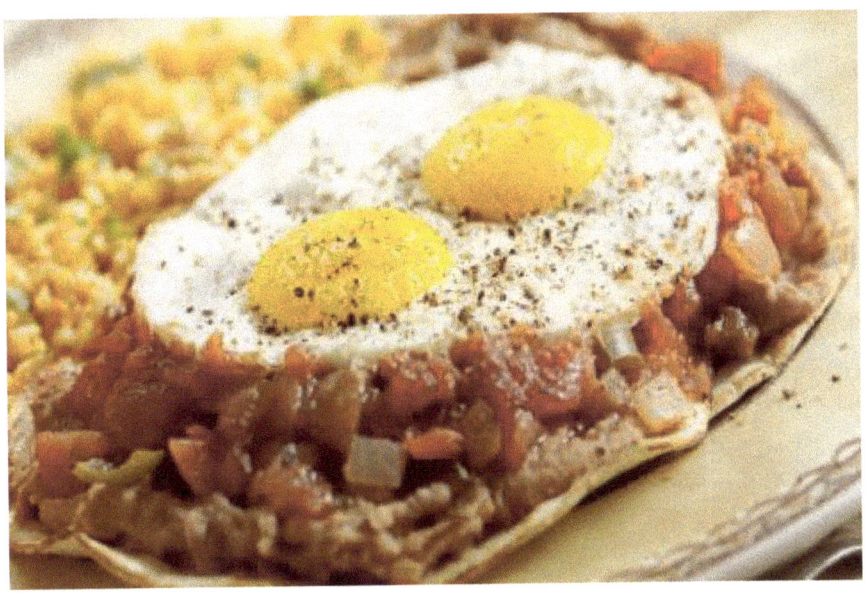

Mediterranean Frittata

Preparing this recipe ahead of time makes for a quick, flavorful meal. Inspired by Italian flavors, this open-faced omelet is loaded with vegetables and herbs and can be enjoyed any time of day. Dried herbs can always be substituted with fresh. Just use a little extra. For added depth, try experimenting with different salts.

Ingredients

7 eggs

$2/3$ cup unsweetened almond milk, coconut milk, or non-fat milk

1 tsp. dried oregano (plus more for garnish)

$3/4$ tsp. dried basil

$1/2$ tsp. salt

Freshly ground black pepper, to taste

2 Tbsp. olive oil

1 clove garlic, minced

2 cups baby spinach

1 (14 oz.) can artichoke hearts in water, well-drained and coarsely chopped

(Remove tough outer layers when chopping; if using marinated artichokes, omit the olive oil and use their marinade oil instead)

$1/2$ cup sliced and pitted Kalamata olives

2 tomatoes, thinly sliced

Instructions

Preheat oven to broil.

In a large bowl, whisk together the eggs, milk, oregano, basil, salt, and pepper until well combined. Set aside.

Heat olive oil in a 10-inch cast-iron skillet over medium heat, coating the surface evenly. Add garlic, spinach, artichoke hearts, and olives. Cover and cook for about 2 minutes, or until the spinach wilts.

Remove the cover, stir the vegetables, and pour the beaten egg mixture over them.

Arrange the tomato slices on top and sprinkle with a little more oregano.

Cook for about 15 minutes, or until the edges are set but the center remains slightly unset

Transfer the skillet to the oven and broil for 3–4 minutes, or until the center is fully set and the top begins to brown. Watch carefully to avoid overcooking.

Remove from the oven, let cool slightly, and serve warm

Greens and Leeks Omelet

YIELD: 1 SERVING

Leeks have a delicate, mild onion flavor that pairs perfectly with nutrient-rich greens. just remember to wash them thoroughly to remove any grit. this omelet is full of fiber, flavor, and wholesome nutrients.

INGREDIENTS

2 tsp. olive oil
¼ cup collard greens, kale, and spinach, stemmed and finely chopped
¼ cup leek, finely chopped
1 tbsp. water
½ tsp. salt
½ tsp. freshly ground black pepper
additional salt and pepper, to taste
2-3 eggs

INSTRUCTIONS

Heat the olive oil in a 12-inch nonstick skillet over medium heat.

Add the greens, leeks, and 1 tbsp. water. cover and cook for 2 minutes.

Uncover and continue cooking, stirring occasionally, until the vegetables are tender, about 2-4 minutes.

While the vegetables are cooking, whisk together the eggs, salt, pepper, and 1 tbsp. water in a small bowl until lightly beaten.

When the vegetables are tender, increase the heat to medium-high for 1 minute.

Pour the eggs evenly over the vegetables and let sit, undisturbed, for 1 minute.

Using a spatula, gently lift one side of the omelet and fold it over the other half.

Cook for about 30 seconds, then flip once more and cook to your desired doneness.

Serve warm and enjoy.

Veggie Style Sausage Hash

YIELD: 4 SERVINGS

A healthy hash that uses veggies instead of potatoes. Healthy and tasty! Who could ask for more? The sausage will cook quicker if it is sliced thin. Choose organic low fat chicken or turkey sausage.

Ingredients

Organic Coconut Oil Spray
4 4-oz. Italian Turkey or Chicken Sausages
1 pint Cherry Tomatoes, halved
1 c.Peppers, diced
1 c. of Broccoli florets
1 Large Zucchini, diced
1 tsp. Dried Oregano
1 tsp. Dried Basil
1 tsp. Garlic Salt or to taste
Freshly Ground Pepper, to taste
1/4 tsp. Red Pepper Flakes, optional (this adds a nice kick or serve with Tabasco Sauce)

Instructions

Preheat oven to 350.
Spray organic t oil evenly over the bottom of a casserole dish.

Slice the sausage and spread out in the pan.

Add broccoli, peppers and zucchini.

Top with tomatoes and sprinkle with oregano, basil and garlic.

Season to taste with garlic salt, ground pepper and red pepper flakes, (if using).

Spray organic olive oil over all, toss and bake for 20 minutes or until all vegetables are tender and sausage is cooked through.

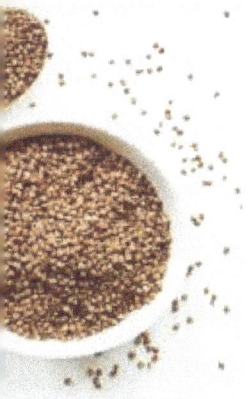

Buckwheat Blueberry Pancakes

(Vegan, Sugar-Free)

Ingredients

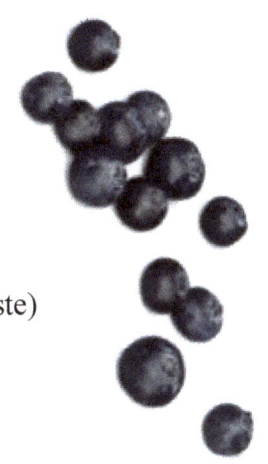

1 cup organic buckwheat flour

1 tsp baking powder

½ tsp cinnamon (optional)

½ tsp vanilla paste

½ tsp powdered Stevia or 10-20 drops blueberry-flavored Stevia (to taste)

1 tbsp flaxseed meal + 3 tbsp water (flax egg substitute)

¾ cup coconut milk, water, or unsweetened almond milk

1 tbsp olive oil or melted coconut oil

½ cup fresh or frozen blueberries

Instructions

Prepare the Flax Egg: In a small bowl, mix flaxseed meal with 3 tbsp water. Let it sit for 5 minutes until it thickens.

Mix Dry Ingredients: In a large bowl, whisk together buckwheat flour, baking powder, cinnamon, and Stevia.

Combine Wet Ingredients: Add the flax egg, non-dairy milk, vanilla, and oil. Stir until the batter is smooth.

Fold in Blueberries: Gently stir in the blueberries.

Cook the Pancakes: Heat a non-stick skillet over medium heat. Pour about ¼ cup of batter for each pancake. Cook until bubbles appear on the surface, then flip and cook for another 1-2 minutes until golden brown.

Serve: Enjoy warm with extra blueberries, a drizzle of Stevia-sweetened fruit compote, or a touch of coconut oil.

Flavor Variations

Apple-Cinnamon Buckwheat Pancakes

Replace blueberries with ½ cup finely chopped Pink Lady apples.

Add ¼ tsp extra cinnamon and a pinch of freshly grated nutmeg.

Raspberry-Lemon Buckwheat Pancakes

Use ½ cup fresh or frozen raspberries instead of blueberries.

Add 1 tsp freshly grated lemon zest.

Cranberry-Orange Buckwheat Pancakes

Substitute ½ cup chopped fresh or frozen cranberries.

Add 1 tsp orange zest for a refreshing twist.

Cherry-Vanilla Buckwheat Pancakes

Use ½ cup pitted and chopped tart or sweet cherries.

Increase vanilla paste to 1 tsp for extra depth and sweetness.

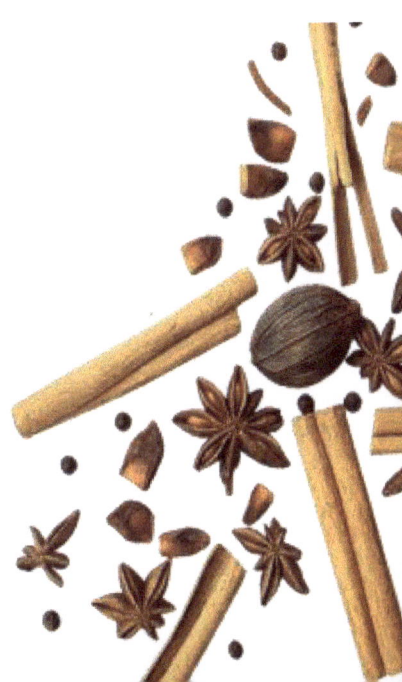

Smoked Salmon With Eggs

The omega-3s in this wild salmon will start your day off right. packed with protein, healthy fats, and nutrients, this hearty breakfast will keep you comfortably full until lunch.

INGREDIENTS

2 tsp. olive oil *or* 1 tsp. ghee

2-3 eggs

Salt and freshly ground black pepper, to taste

3 oz. roasted wild salmon

2 roasted red pepper halves, prepared
¼ avocado, thinly sliced

4 thin red onion rings

INSTRUCTIONS

PREPARE THE SALMON: Preheat oven to 350°f (175°c). season the salmon with salt and pepper. Bake for about 10 minutes, or until the fillet flakes easily with a fork.

COOK THE EGGS: Heat olive oil (or ghee) in a large skillet over medium heat. Carefully crack the eggs. Season lightly with salt and pepper, and cook to your preference, sunny-side up, over easy, over medium, or even soft-boiled.

ASSEMBLE THE PLATE: Place the cooked eggs on a plate. layer with roasted salmon, red pepper halves, avocado slices, and onion rings.

Serve warm and enjoy a nutrient–dense start to your day.

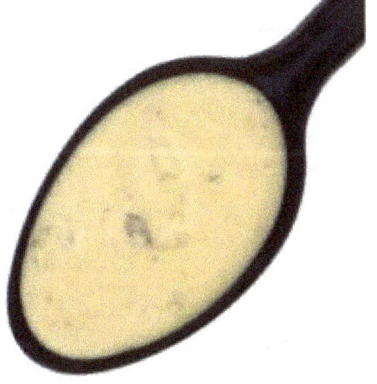

Soups

Soup is one of the most comforting and nourishing foods you can enjoy. It's easy to digest, gentle on the stomach, and provides essential vitamins, minerals, and hydration, all of which are especially important during treatment and recovery.

Because of its warm, soothing nature, soup can help calm nausea, ease digestive issues, and encourage better hydration. Its aroma and taste can also stimulate appetite, which is often a challenge during illness or treatment. By combining a variety of vegetables, lean proteins such as chicken, fish, or beans, and whole grains, soups can deliver a powerful mix of nutrients and fiber to support overall health.

Some vegetables commonly used in soups include:

Tomatoes – rich in lycopene, a strong antioxidant
Cruciferous vegetables like broccoli and cauliflower, linked to potential cancer-fighting benefits
Beans and legumes – packed with plant-based protein and fiber
Soups are also highly versatile: they can be blended smoothly for easy consumption, kept chunky for a hearty meal, or prepared as broth-based dishes for a lighter option.

For the healthiest choice, opt for broth-based soups instead of creamy varieties, which may be higher in fat. Load them with fiber-rich vegetables, fresh herbs, and lean proteins to create meals that are not only delicious but also deeply nourishing.

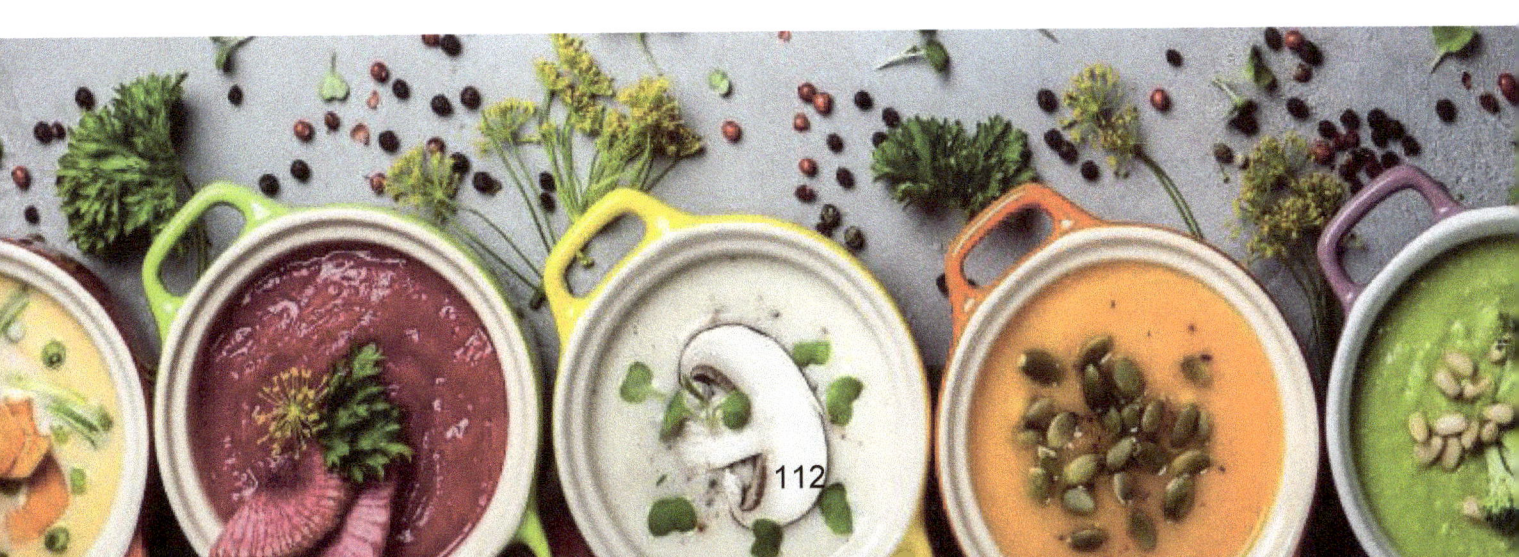

Chicken Soup

YIELD: 4 SERVINGS

Who doesn't love a bowl of chicken soup? This quick version is packed with flavor and nourishing vegetables, and it can be made start to finish in under 10 minutes!

Ingredients

2 Tbsp. extra-virgin olive oil (EVOO)
1 onion, chopped
2-3 garlic cloves, minced
1 Tbsp. fresh ginger, minced
4 Cups oflow-sodium chicken broth
1-2 cups zucchini, thinly sliced
½ cup celery, chopped
½ cup carrots, shredded
1 cup kale, cut into bite-size pieces
2 Cups broccoli florets
2 Cups of cauliflower florets
2 Cups cooked chicken, shredded or diced
¼ cup fresh basil leaves, sliced
½ cup parsley, chopped, bay leaf
1 avocado, sliced (for topping)

Instructions

Heat a large stockpot over medium heat. Add the olive oil, onion, garlic, and ginger. Cook 1-2 minutes, stirring often, until the onion softens.

Add the chicken broth, zucchini, celery, carrots, parsley, broccoli, cauliflower, and the bay leaf. Cook 2-3 minutes, until the vegetables are just tender.

Stir in the chicken, basil, and kale. Simmer for 10-20 minutes, allowing the flavors to blend. Remove the bay leaf before serving. Ladle into bowls and top with avocado slices.

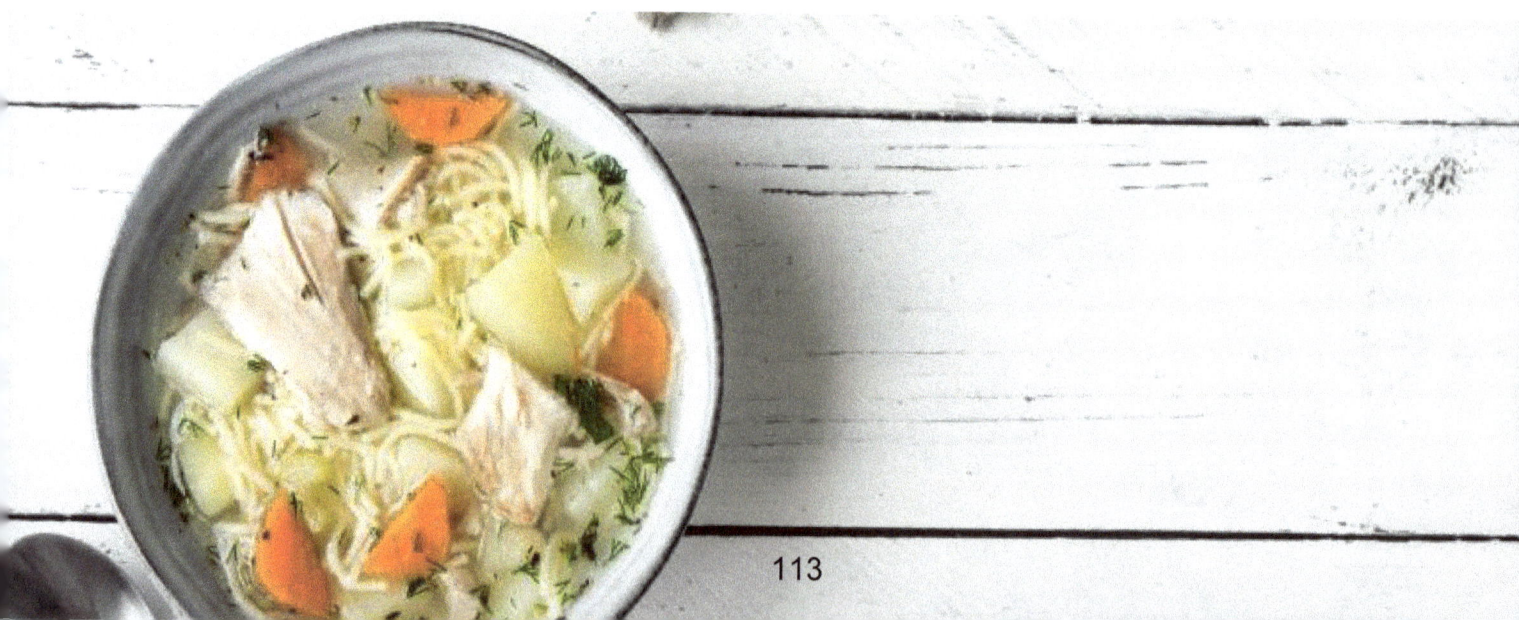

Spicy Cabbage Soup

A hearty, flavor-packed soup loaded with nutrient-rich vegetables and warming spices. Anti-inflammatory ingredients like turmeric and cumin make this not only delicious but also deeply healing.

Ingredients

1 Tbsp. olive oil

1 large onion, diced

3 cloves garlic, minced

1 cup carrots, sliced

1 cup broccoli florets

2 cups cabbage, thinly sliced

1 can (14 oz.) diced tomatoes (no salt added)

4 cups organic vegetable broth

1 Tbsp. tomato paste

1 tsp. cumin

1 tsp. smoked chili flakes or cayenne (adjust to heat preference)

½ tsp. turmeric (anti-inflammatory boost)

½ tsp. ground coriander

1 tsp. paprika

½ tsp. dried thyme *or* oregano

Salt and freshly ground black pepper, to taste

Juice of ½ lemon (for a fresh finish)

½ cup fresh cilantro *or* parsley, chopped (for garnish)

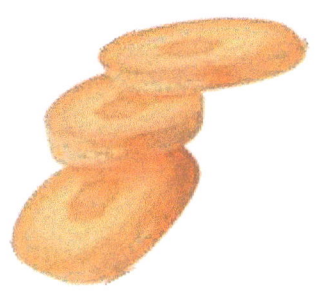

Instructions

Heat olive oil in a large pot over medium heat.

Add the onion and cook for 3-4 minutes, until softened.

Stir in garlic, cumin, chili flakes, turmeric, coriander, paprika, and thyme.

Cook for 1 minute, until fragrant.

Build the flavor base: Add carrots and cabbage, stirring well to coat with the spices.

Pour in the diced tomatoes, tomato paste, and vegetable broth. Bring to a gentle simmer.

Cook for about 15 minutes, then add the broccoli.

Simmer for another 5-7 minutes, until all vegetables are tender but not mushy.

Stir in the lemon juice and adjust the seasoning with salt and black pepper.

Garnish with fresh cilantro or parsley and serve hot.

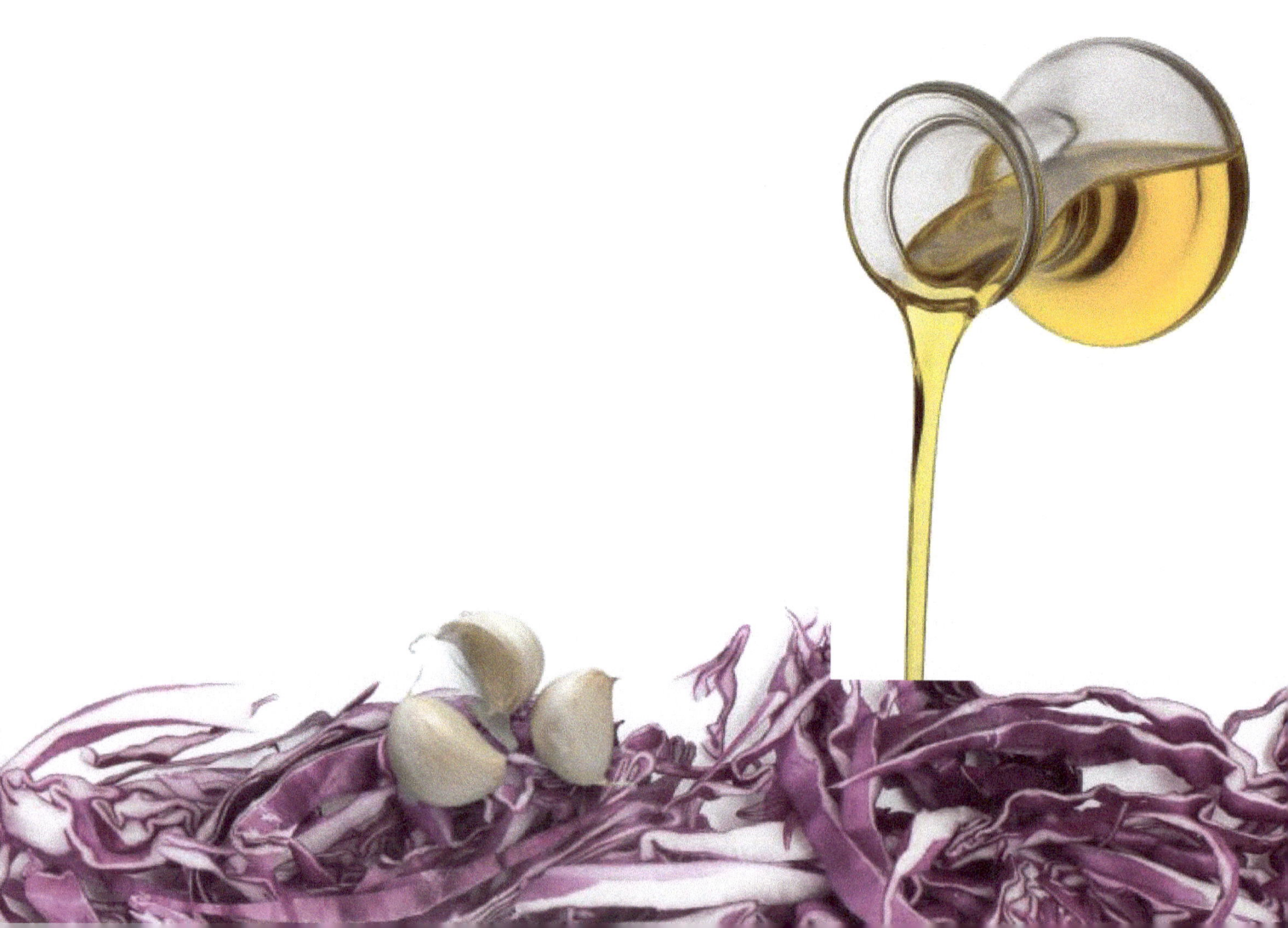

Turkey Soup

A nourishing way to use fresh or leftover turkey, this soup is packed with vegetables, rich flavor, and wholesome black rice. Perfect for a cozy, nutrient-dense meal.

Ingredients

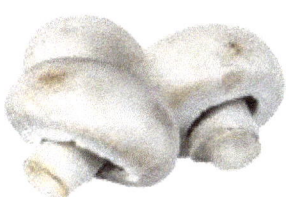

1-2 cups roasted or poached turkey breast or thighs (or leftover turkey, lightly shredded or diced)
Broth from turkey (if poached) or turkey broth from a crock pot recipe
1 onion, diced
1 clove garlic, minced
½ cup green beans, snapped
1 large carrot, sliced
1 cup mushrooms, sliced
½ cup black rice
3-4 cups organic turkey broth (adjust as needed)
1 Tbsp. walnut oil, flaxseed oil, or ghee
½ tsp. dried thyme
Fresh parsley, chopped, for garnish

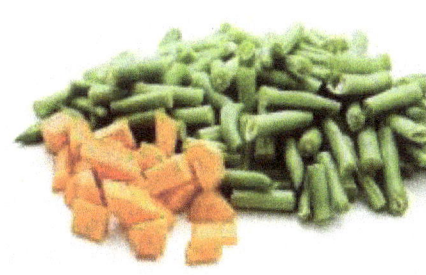

Instructions

In a large stock pot, heat the oil over medium heat.
Add the onion and cook until lightly browned, about 5-7 minutes. Stir in the garlic and cook another 2-3 minutes. *(This step builds flavor.)*
Add the mushrooms and cook for 1-2 minutes, then add the remaining vegetables one at a time, lightly cooking each before adding the next.
Stir in the turkey, mixing well with the vegetables.
Pour in the broth (add extra if needed to ensure enough liquid for the rice to cook and still leave broth for the soup).
Bring to a light boil, then stir in the rice.
Reduce the heat to a simmer, cover, and cook according to the rice package directions, adding broth as needed.
Season with thyme, adjust salt and pepper if desired, and garnish with fresh parsley before serving.

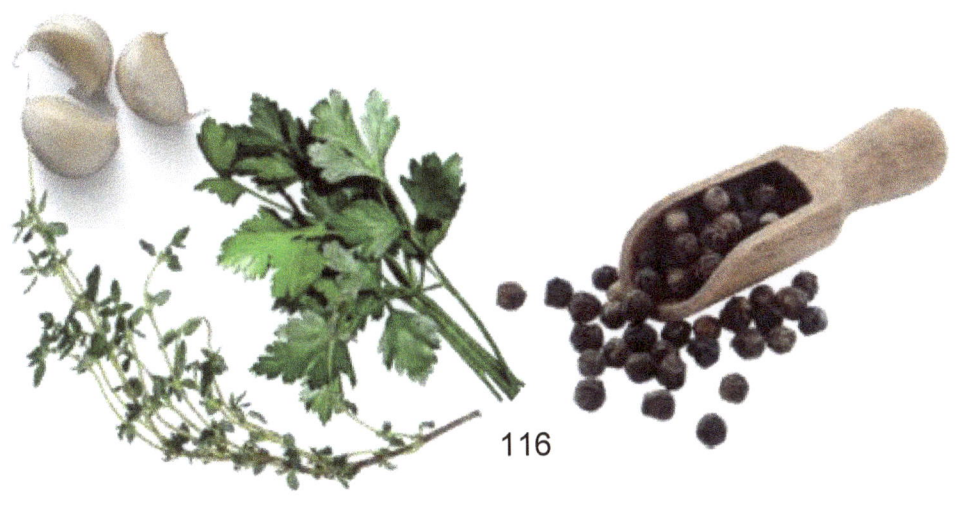

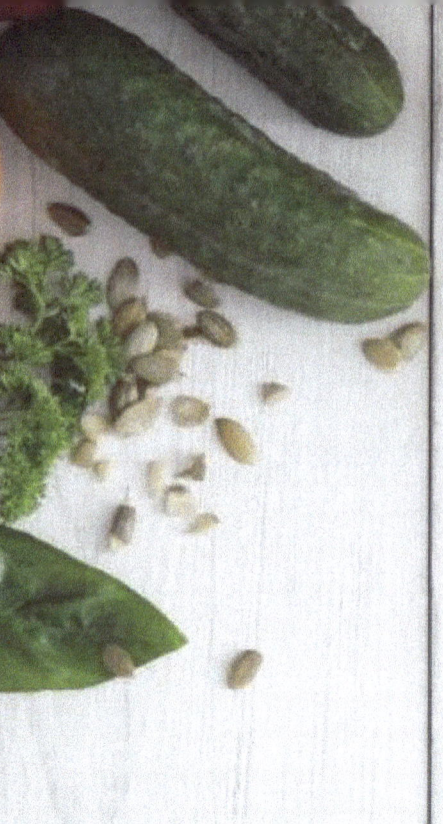

Harvest Soup

One of the tastiest soups you'll ever have.
It warms you up on a cool day
and provides a powerhouse of nutrients.

Ingredients

Extra-virgin olive oil
8 carrots, peeled and sliced
1 large onion, diced
2-3 celery hearts with leaves, chopped
1 clove garlic, crushed and diced
1 small head of broccoli, chopped
1 cup peas (fresh or frozen)
2 cups green beans, chopped
1 red pepper, diced
1 tsp. dried thyme
1 tsp. dried basil
1 bay leaf
1 tsp. salt (or to taste)
1 tsp. black pepper (or to taste)
1-2 cartons organic vegetable broth
1 (32 oz.) can strained tomatoes

Instructions

In a large stock pot, heat a drizzle of olive oil over medium heat.
Add the onion, carrots, and celery. Sauté until they begin to soften, about 4 minutes.
Add broccoli, red pepper, cauliflower (if using), garlic, and peas.
Add more olive oil as needed to prevent sticking.
Pour in the vegetable broth, strained tomatoes,
and add the thyme, basil, bay leaf, salt, and pepper. Bring to a light boil.
Reduce the heat to a simmer and taste, adjusting seasonings as needed.
Cook slowly for at least 3-4 hours, stirring occasionally to prevent sticking.
The longer it simmers, the richer and more blended the flavors become.

Meatball Minestrone Soup

YIELD: 3 SERVINGS

Mini meatballs take the place of pasta or beans in this twist on classic minestrone. Grass-fed ground turkey is rich in Omega-3s and has a deeper, richer flavor compared to corn-fed turkey. If you buy ground turkey by the pound, freeze the extra ½ pound and save it to make this soup again another time.

Ingredients

For the Mini Meatballs

1 lb. lean ground turkey

4 mushrooms, grated or finely chopped

2 Tbsp. ground flax

¼ cup fresh basil, chopped

1 egg

¼ tsp. salt

¼ tsp. freshly ground black pepper

2 Tbsp. olive oil

For the Soup

½ yellow or red onion, chopped

2 garlic cloves, minced

1 (15 oz.) can diced tomatoes

1 tsp. oregano

2 cups broccoli florets

2 cups cauliflower florets

½ cup carrot, grated

32 oz. organic chicken or vegetable broth

Instructions

Prepare the meatballs: In a large bowl, combine the ground turkey, mushrooms, ground flax, basil, egg, salt, and pepper. Mix well.

Form into ½-inch meatballs and set aside on a plate.

Heat a large stockpot over medium heat and add the olive oil.

Add the meatballs and cook for 2-3 minutes, turning occasionally, until lightly browned.

Add the onion and garlic around the meatballs. Stir gently and cook until softened, 1-2 minutes.

Stir in the diced tomatoes and oregano.

Cook for another 1-2 minutes to build flavor.

Add the broccoli, cauliflower, carrots, and broth. Stir to combine.

Bring to a simmer over medium heat and cook for 5-6 minutes, until the broccoli is tender and the meatballs are cooked through.

Taste and adjust with additional salt and pepper if needed.

Serving Suggestion

This soup is especially delicious served over barley cooked in organic turkey broth with fresh basil stirred in for extra flavor.

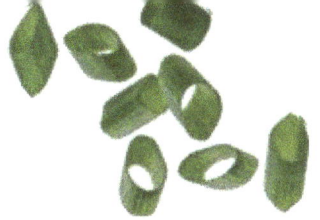

Onions & Cancer Prevention

Mechanistic studies provide compelling evidence that garlic, onions, and their sulfur compounds can influence tumor biology, alter the tumor microenvironment, affect precancerous cells, and ultimately help decrease cancer risk.

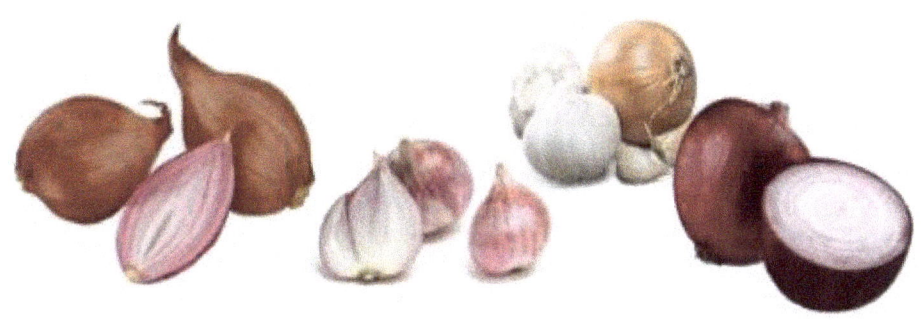

According to a study led by Dr. Rui Hai Liu, M.D., Ph.D., associate professor of food science at Cornell University, varieties such as shallots, Western Yellow, pungent yellow, and Northern Red onions contain some of the highest levels of anti-cancer compounds among those tested.

"Onions are one of the richest sources of flavonoids in the human diet," Dr. Liu explains. "They are not only anti-cancer, but also anti-bacterial, anti-viral, anti-allergenic, and anti-inflammatory."

Researchers now estimate that about one-third of cancer cases could be prevented through diet alone, a powerful reminder of the role food plays in our health and longevity.

Choose foods like onions and garlic that nourish your body, strengthen your immune system, and fight cancer cell growth naturally.

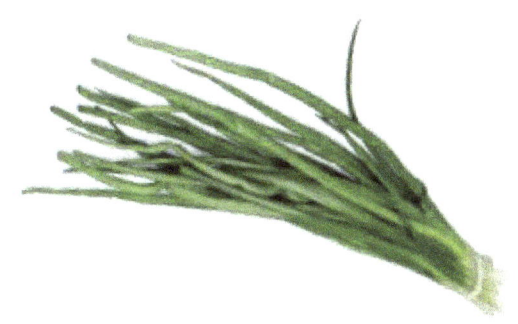

French Onion & Mushroom Soup
Dairy Free

YIELD: 4 SERVINGS

This nourishing soup is warm, rich, and full of deep umami flavors from slow-cooked onions and earthy mushrooms.

Ingredients

2 Large yellow onions, thinly sliced

1 red onion, thinly sliced,
2 shallots, thinly sliced
1 cup organic mushrooms (cremini or shiitake), sliced

2 Tbsp. organic olive oil

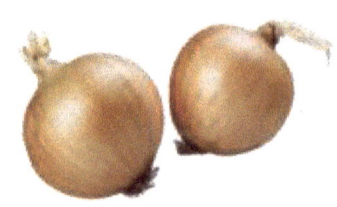

2 Cloves, organic garlic, minced

4 cups organic low-sodium vegetable broth (or water)
½ tsp. black pepper

½ tsp. dried thyme
1 bay leaf
1 Tbsp. balsamic vinegar (optional, for depth of flavor)

Instructions

Caramelize the onions: In a large pot, heat the olive oil over medium-low heat. Add the yellow onions, red onions, and shallots. Cook slowly, stirring occasionally, for 20-30 minutes, until deeply golden and caramelized.

Add garlic & mushrooms: Stir in the garlic and mushrooms.

Cook for another 5-10 minutes, until softened and lightly browned.

Simmer: Pour in the vegetable broth, then add black pepper, thyme, and the bay leaf. Simmer for 20-30 minutes to allow flavors to develop.

Finish & serve: Remove the bay leaf, stir in balsamic vinegar (if using), and adjust seasoning to taste. Serve hot.

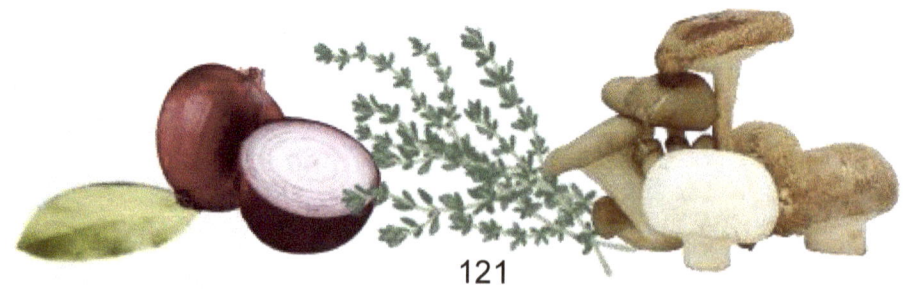

Creamy Butternut Squash Soup

One of my very favorite soups! Creamy, cozy, and packed with flavor, perfect for a nourishing

meal on a chilly day.

Ingredients

1 medium butternut squash, peeled and cubed

1 small onion, chopped

2 cloves garlic, minced

2 Tbsp. olive oil

4 cups low-sodium organic vegetable broth

½ tsp. black pepper

¼ tsp. ground nutmeg

½ cup unsweetened coconut milk

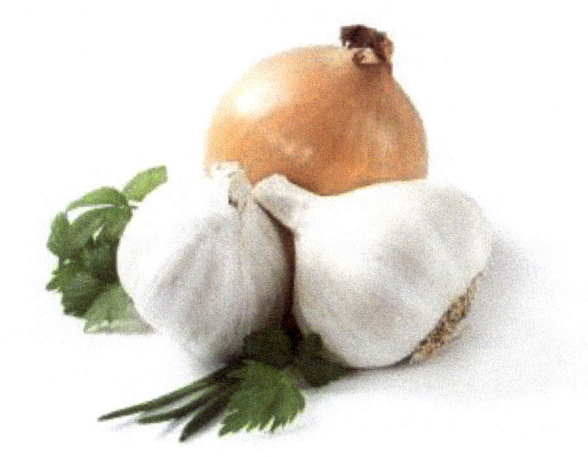

Instructions

Prepare the squash: For easy prep, pierce the butternut squash in several places with a knife and place it on a parchment-lined baking pan. Bake at 375°F for 30-45 minutes, until just softened. Let it cool, then peel, remove the seeds, and cube.

Tip: You can do this a day ahead, refrigerate and cube later.

Sauté the aromatics: Heat olive oil in a large pot over medium heat. Add onion and garlic, cooking until softened and fragrant.

Build the soup: Add cubed squash, black pepper, nutmeg, and vegetable broth. Bring to a boil, then reduce to a simmer. Cook for about 20 minutes, or until the squash is very tender.

Make it creamy: Stir in the coconut milk. Using an immersion blender (or carefully transferring to a regular blender), puree until smooth and creamy.

Serve: Ladle into bowls and garnish with pumpkin seeds for a crunchy, nutritious finish. Serve warm.

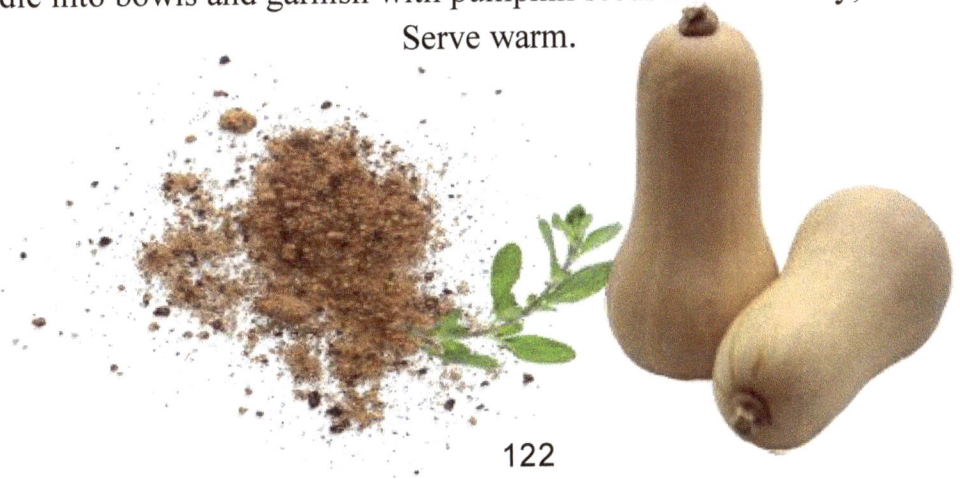

Sugar And Breast Cancer Risk

Eating large amounts of desserts and sweets may increase the risk of breast cancer, particularly for premenopausal women. These foods are often high in calories, refined carbohydrates, and saturated fats, all of which can negatively impact health.

Why This Matters:

Insulin Resistance

Consuming too much sugar or foods with a high glycemic index can lead to insulin resistance. This, in turn, increases insulin-related growth factors that may promote the development of breast cancer.

Ovarian Steroid Secretion

Excess insulin can stimulate the ovaries to produce estrogen and androgens, both of which have been linked to an increased risk of breast cancer.

Poor Nutrient Content

Desserts and sweet foods are often nutrient-poor but calorie-dense, containing high levels of refined carbohydrates and saturated fats. These can contribute to inflammation, weight gain, and metabolic changes that may support cancer growth.

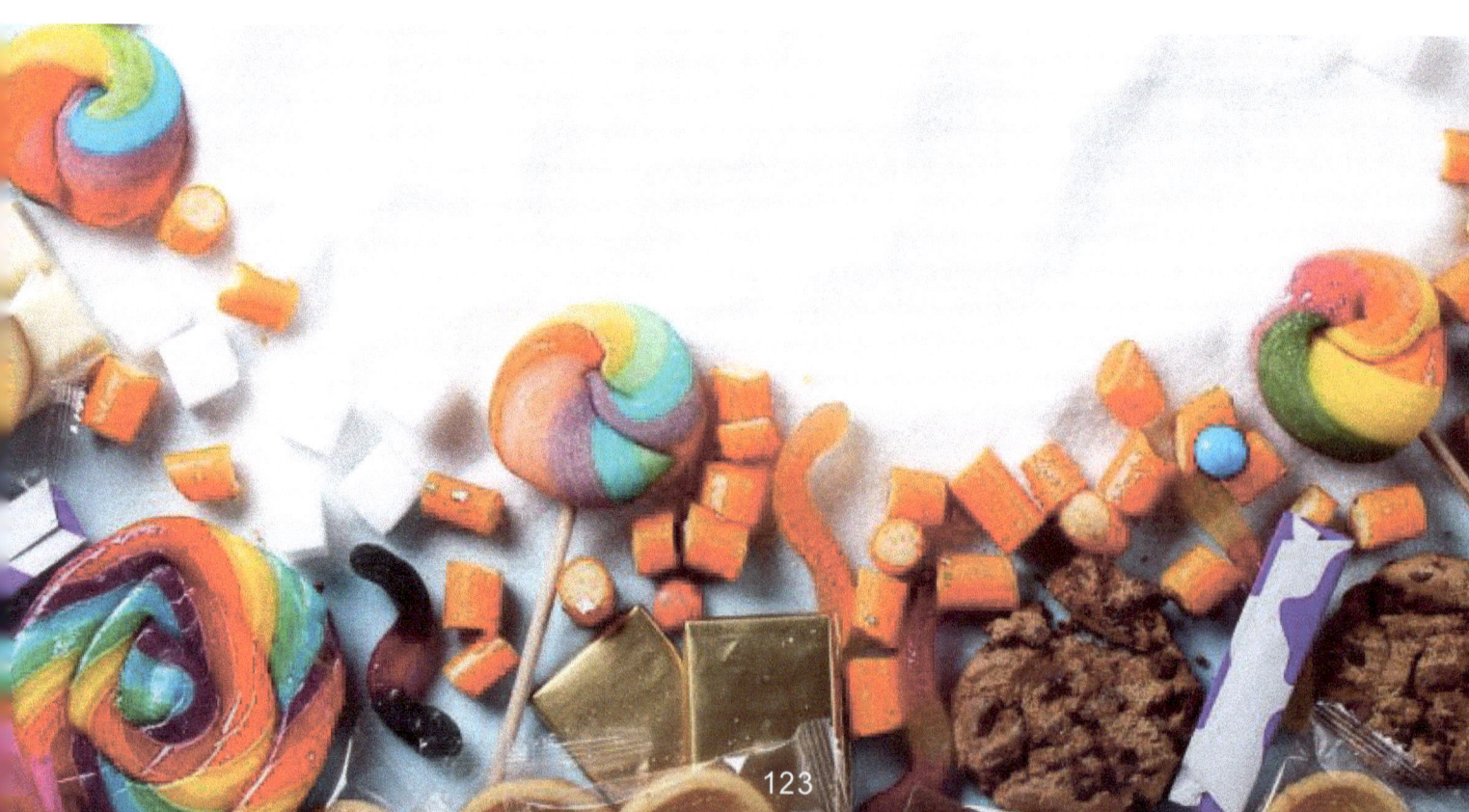

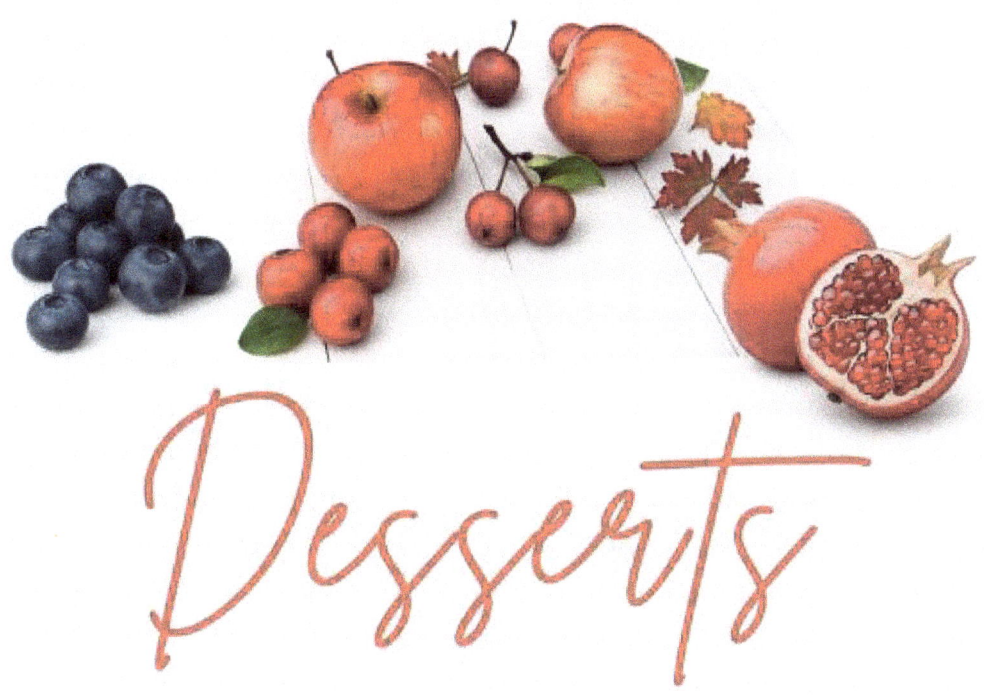

Desserts

Eating the right foods can make a powerful difference when facing breast cancer, and that includes choosing smart fruits and low-sugar snacks. These foods are packed with essential vitamins, minerals, and antioxidants that help support your body, reduce inflammation, and keep your energy steady.

The natural sweetness of fresh fruit satisfies cravings without causing the sharp sugar spikes that processed snacks often bring. Pairing fruit with nuts or seeds adds healthy fats and protein, helping you stay full, energized, and balanced throughout the day.

When nausea or fatigue makes full meals unappealing, small, nutrient-dense snacks are the perfect solution. They deliver nourishment in gentle, manageable portions, giving your body exactly what it needs without overwhelming your system. Think of them as little boosts of strength, simple, tasty, and effective.

Remember: Big flavor doesn't have to come with big sugar. The less added sugar you eat, the better. Since cancer cells thrive on sugar, limiting it is one of the most important steps you can take to protect your health. All while still enjoying delicious, nourishing foods.

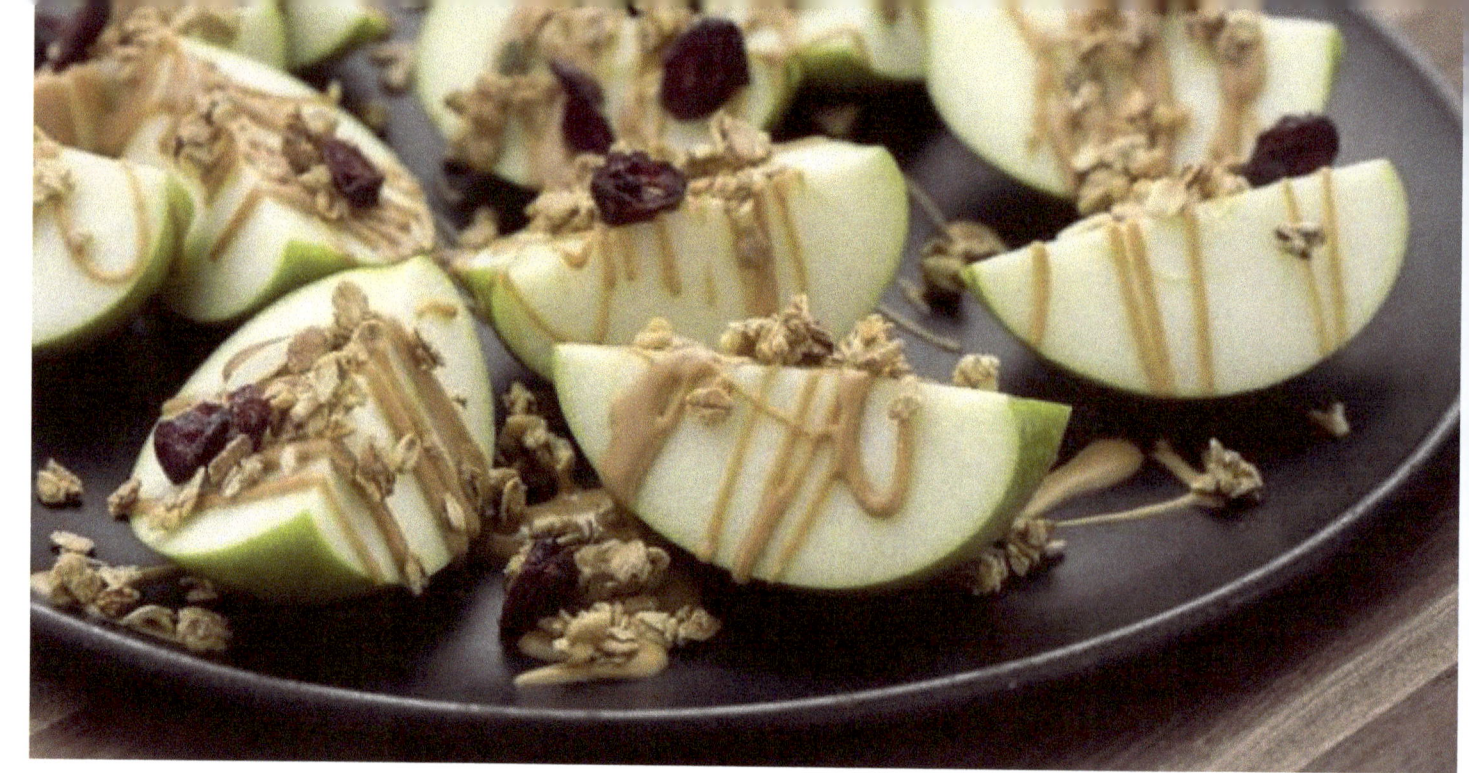

Apple Nachos

A crunchy, sweet, and satisfying treat, perfect when you're craving dessert but want to keep it light and nourishing.

Ingredients

1-3 apples, cut into thin slices

¼ cup PB2 powder (lower in fat)

½ cup Greek yogurt, mixed with stevia (flavor of choice)

2 Tbsp. mini dark chocolate chips

¼ cup crushed nuts (almonds, walnuts, or pecans)

Directions

Arrange the apple slices neatly on a plate or platter.

Mix the PB2 powder with water until smooth, then stir it into the Greek yogurt and stevia mixture.

Drizzle the yogurt-peanut butter mixture over the apple slices with a spoon.

Sprinkle mini dark chocolate chips and crushed nuts evenly over the apples.

Serve immediately and enjoy!

Health Note

Although chocolate tastes so good, remember that moderation matters. Sugar can feed cancer cells, so stick with the small amount called for in this recipe. Avoid adding more.

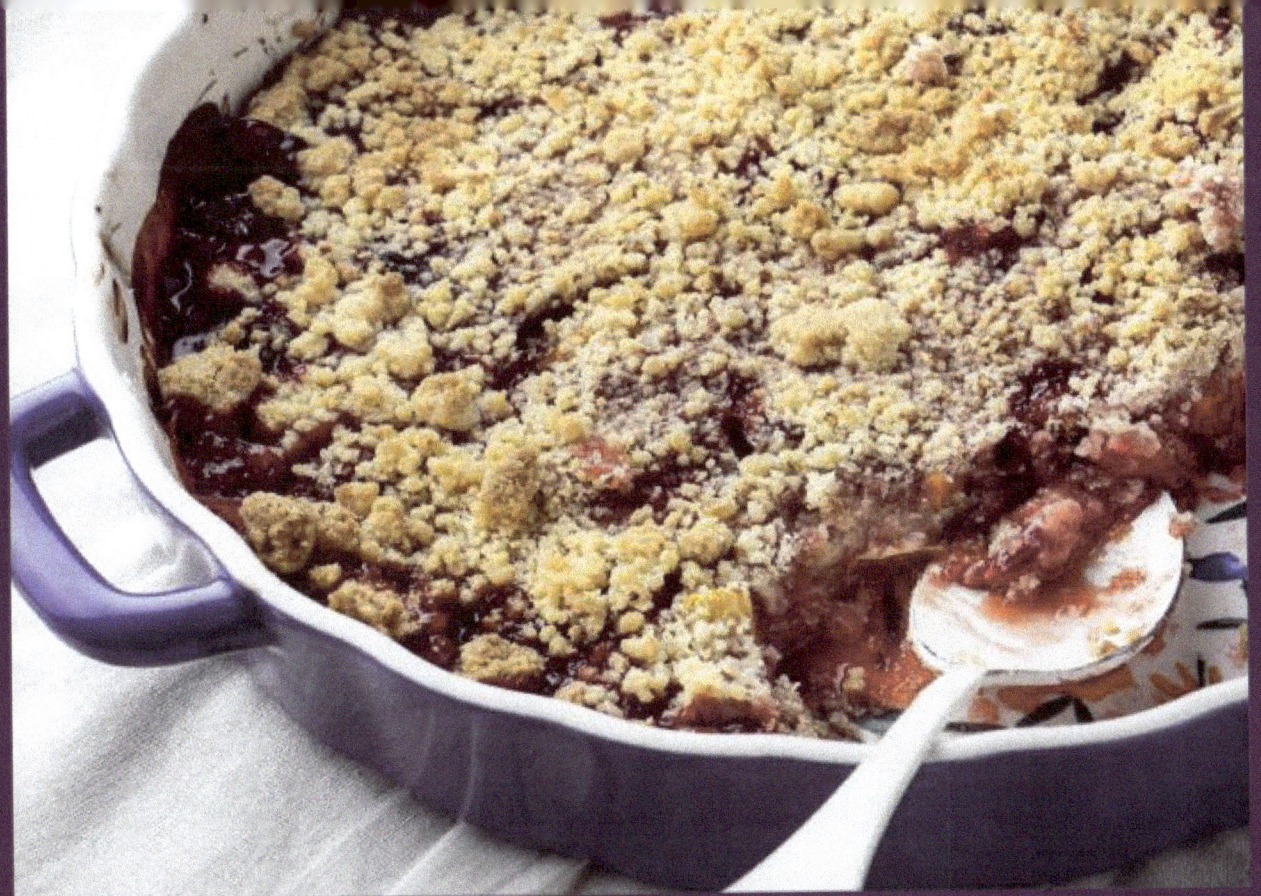

Berry Crumble

YIELD: 4 SERVINGS

Ingredients

3 cups berries (cherries or your choice)

1 tbsp finely chopped crystallized ginger

¼ cup organic non-GMO flour

For the crumble:

½ cup chopped walnuts

½ cup chopped pecans **For the garnish:**

½ cup nonfat Greek yogurt
2 tbsp organic maple syrup

½ cup chopped pistachios

½ cup organic rolled oats

¼ cup organic non-GMO flour

½ tsp cinnamon

½ tsp nutmeg

¼ tsp salt

2 tbsp organic cold-pressed coconut oil

20 drops toffee stevia (or sweetener of choice)

1 tsp vanilla bean paste

For the garnish:

½ cup nonfat Greek yogurt
2 tbsp organic maple syrup

Directions

- **Prepare the berries:** Wash the berries and gently pat dry with a paper towel. Place them in a bowl, sprinkle with flour, and toss to coat.

- **Assemble the filling:** Grease a 9x9-inch pan with coconut oil spray. Place the berries in the pan, leaving excess flour in the bowl. Sprinkle with the crystallized ginger.

- **Make the crumble:** In a bowl, combine the walnuts, pecans, pistachios, oats, flour, cinnamon, and nutmeg. In a small bowl, mix together the coconut oil, maple syrup, stevia, and vanilla. Pour the wet mixture over the dry ingredients and mix well.

- **Top and bake:** Evenly spread the nut mixture over the berries and ginger. Bake in a preheated oven at 350°F (175°C) for about 30 minutes, or until bubbly. If using frozen fruit, bake for about 45 minutes.

- **Finish with garnish:** Mix the Greek yogurt with maple syrup.

- Garnish each serving with a dollop of the yogurt mixture.

126

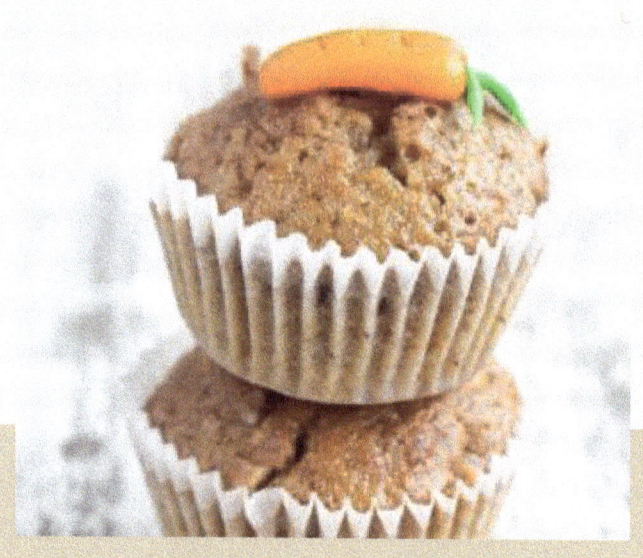

Sweet Moist Breakfast Muffins

INGREDIENTS

¾ cup cooked organic mashed sweet potato (about one)

¼ cup grated organic carrot (about one small carrot)

½ cup grated organic apple (about half of an apple)

½ cup grated unsweetened organic coconut

½ cup dried organic sour cherries

¼ cup finely chopped organic dried figs

½ cup finely chopped nuts (walnuts, pecans, hazelnuts, your choice)

¾ cup almond flour

1 ¼ tsp cinnamon

⅛ cup organic pure maple syrup

1 tsp baking powder

2 organic eggs

¼ tsp freshly grated nutmeg

DIRECTIONS

Preheat oven to 350°F.

In a large bowl, combine all ingredients and mix slowly if using an electric mixer.

Divide batter into muffin cups (use the paper kind).

Bake for 30 minutes, or until a knife inserted in the center comes out clean and the top is slightly brown.

Remove from oven and cool for 10 minutes before eating.

Makes about nine muffins.

Triple Berry & Cherry Compote

Cherries contain relatively high levels of anthocyanins, flavonoids responsible for their deep red color. These compounds are known for their antioxidant, anti-inflammatory, and chemopreventive properties, making this dish both delicious and health-supportive.

This naturally sweet, nutrient-packed compote can be enjoyed on its own or used as a versatile topping.

Ingredients

½ cup fresh or frozen cranberries
½ cup fresh or frozen tart cherries (pitted)
½ cup fresh or frozen raspberries ¼ cup pomegranate juice
½ tsp. grated ginger
½ tsp. vanilla paste
½-1 tsp. powdered stevia or 10-20 drops cranberry stevia (adjust to taste)

Instructions

In a small saucepan over medium heat, combine cranberries, cherries, raspberries, and pomegranate juice.

Bring to a gentle simmer and cook for 10-15 minutes, stirring occasionally, until the fruit softens and releases its juices.

Mash lightly with a spoon or fork to your preferred texture, chunky or smooth.

Stir in grated ginger, vanilla paste, and stevia. Adjust sweetness carefully, as stevia is very concentrated.

Let cool slightly before serving.

Ways to Enjoy

Serve warm or chilled as a light dessert.
Top with walnuts or sprinkle with whole organic oats for added crunch.
Spread on whole-grain toast.
Drizzle over buckwheat pancakes or waffles.
Stir into Greek yogurt or oatmeal for a quick, antioxidant-rich breakfast.

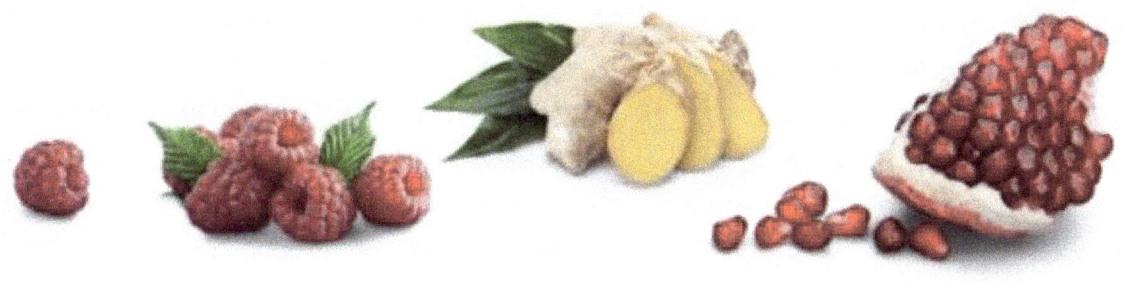

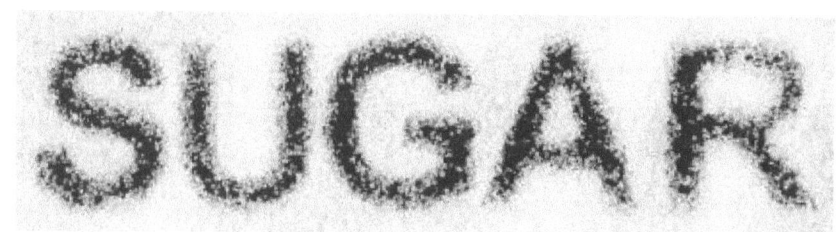

The idea that breast cancer is *"fed by sugar"* is, at best, a partial explanation of the relationship between sugar consumption and breast cancer risk.

When we consume sucrose (sugar), enzymes in the digestive tract break it down into glucose, which is the primary energy source for all of our cells.

Every cell in the body healthy or cancerous, requires glucose to survive. It is true that cancer cells typically consume glucose at a much higher rate than normal cells. Research shows that compounds that block glucose uptake in tumor cells may help inhibit their growth and viability. However, it is important to note that cancer cells can obtain glucose from many dietary sources, not just refined sugar.

How Sugar Promotes Cancer Risk

Sugar plays a direct role in promoting breast cancer beyond simply serving as fuel for cancer cell metabolism. High sugar intake can contribute to insulin resistance and increased circulating insulin, which promotes cancer growth.

Refined carbohydrates and sugary foods often lead to chronic inflammation and oxidative stress, both of which are linked to cancer development.

Diets rich in sweets and processed sugars may displace nutrient-dense foods that help protect against cancer.

Evidence from Case-Control Studies

Japan: A case-control study found that breast cancer risk was positively associated with higher intakes of bread, cake, and soft drinks sweetened with sugar.

Italy: Another study reported that breast cancer risk increased with higher consumption of bread, pasta, and refined sugar.

United States: A U.S. case-control study found that frequent consumption of sweets, especially desserts, was associated with a higher risk of breast cancer.

Mango & Strawberry Walnut Crisp

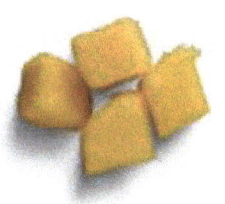

Ingredients

1 cup fresh mango, diced
1 cup fresh strawberries, sliced
½ cup red or black grapes, halved
½ tsp. cinnamon
A light grating of nutmeg
½ tsp. vanilla paste
1 tsp. powdered stevia or 10-20 drops strawberry stevia
½ cup walnuts, chopped
¼ cup unsweetened organic shredded coconut (optional)
1 Tbsp. olive oil or melted coconut oil

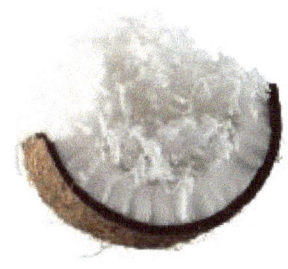

Instructions

Preheat oven to 350°F (175°C).
Mix fruit: In a medium bowl, toss mango, strawberries, grapes, cinnamon, nutmeg, vanilla, and stevia. Spread evenly in a baking dish.
Prepare topping: In another bowl, combine walnuts, shredded coconut (if using), and oil. Mix until crumbly.
Assemble & bake: Sprinkle the walnut mixture evenly over the fruit. Bake for 15-20 minutes, until the fruit softens and the topping is golden.
Serve: Enjoy warm straight from the oven, or chill for a refreshing treat.
Serving Tip: Try topping with a spoonful of nonfat Greek yogurt or a drizzle of organic maple syrup for extra creaminess and flavor.

Chemopreventive means that strawberries may help reduce the risk of cancer returning.

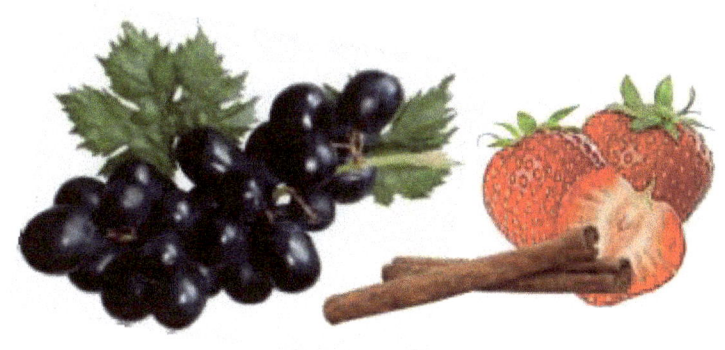

Raspberries, Peaches & Breast Cancer Prevention

Raspberries are a rich source of anthocyanins, plant pigments with powerful chemopreventive properties that also give the berries their deep, vibrant color. The most important anthocyanins found in raspberries include cyanidin, pelargonidin, and malvidin.

In one study, women in the highest quartile of anthocyanin intake had a significantly lower risk of breast cancer compared to those in the lowest quartile. Beyond cancer prevention, anthocyanins have also been shown to help protect the heart by reducing Adriamycin (doxorubicin)-induced cardiotoxicity, a common side effect of certain chemotherapy treatments.

Peaches also play an important role in cancer prevention. Harvard research has linked peach consumption to a reduced risk of certain breast cancers. Additionally, their findings reinforce that eating more fruits and vegetables overall may help lower breast cancer risk while supporting general health and wellness.

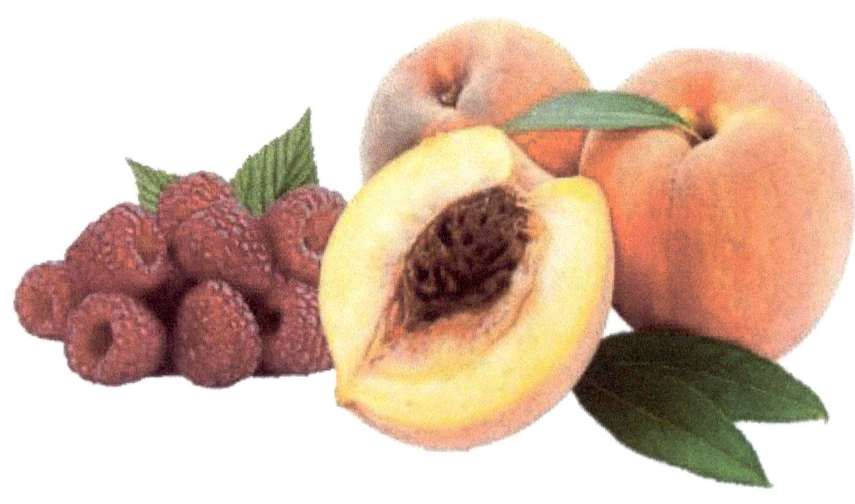

Raspberry, Peach & Orange Parfait With Walnuts (No-Bake, Sugar-Free)

A refreshing, antioxidant–rich fruit parfait with the natural sweetness of berries, peaches, and oranges, balanced by crunchy nuts and seeds. Light, energizing, and nourishing. Perfect as a snack, breakfast, or light dessert.

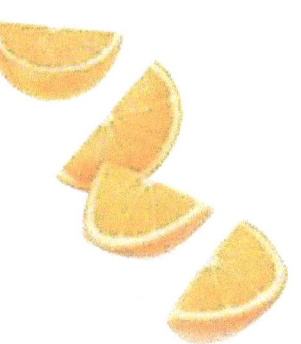

Ingredients

1 cup fresh raspberries

1 ripe peach, diced

1 small orange, segmented and chopped

1 Tbsp. orange zest

1 tsp. stevia (adjust to taste)

½ cup walnuts, chopped

2 Tbsp. unsweetened organic shredded coconut (optional)

2 Tbsp. pumpkin seeds

Coconut milk kefir (optional, for drizzling)

Instructions

Prepare the fruit: In a bowl, gently toss raspberries, diced peach, orange pieces, and orange zest. Sprinkle with stevia and let sit for 5 minutes to allow the flavors to develop.

Make the topping: In a small bowl, combine walnuts, shredded coconut (if using), and pumpkin seeds.

Assemble: Layer the fruit mixture into glasses or bowls. Sprinkle the walnut topping over each serving.

Chill or serve immediately: Enjoy fresh, or refrigerate for 10 minutes to let the flavors blend. For added creaminess, drizzle with coconut milk kefir (sweeten with a touch of stevia if desired).

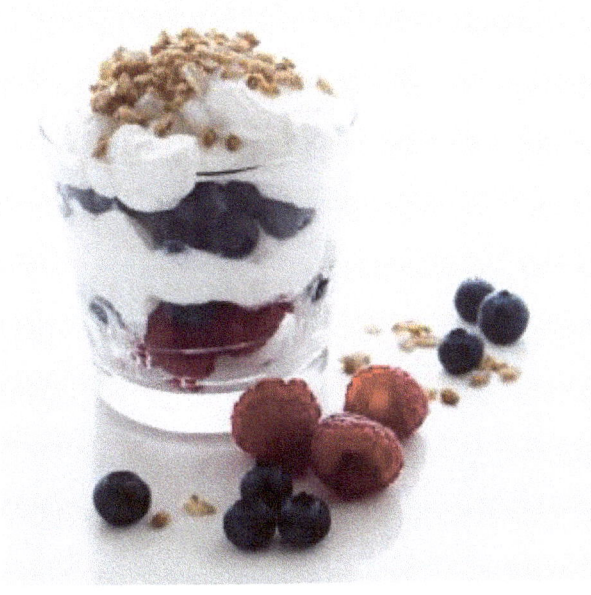

Rich Chocolate Bread

This loaf is excellent for breakfast, perfect as a dessert, wonderful with coffee, or even as a midday snack.
Truly one of my favorite recipes, moist, rich, and full of wholesome flavor.

Ingredients

1 cup grated zucchini (about 1 small zucchini)

¾ cup all-natural almond butter *or* walnut butter (creamy or crunchy)

¼ cup organic pure maple syrup *or* 25 drops of chocolate stevia

2 organic eggs, slightly beaten

½ tsp. organic vanilla paste

2 Tbsp. organic coconut flour *or* almond flour

1 tsp. baking soda

¾ tsp. cinnamon

½ cup dark chocolate (80% or higher cacao), finely chopped

9-12 drops of chocolate stevia

Directions

Preheat oven to 350°F (175°C). Line an 8 x 4-inch loaf pan with parchment paper and lightly spray with extra-virgin olive oil or organic coconut oil.

Mix wet ingredients: In a large bowl, whisk together zucchini, almond butter, maple syrup (or stevia), eggs, and vanilla until well combined and creamy.

Add dry ingredients: Stir in coconut/almond flour, baking soda, and cinnamon until evenly mixed.

Prepare chocolate: In a small bowl, combine chopped dark chocolate with the chocolate stevia drops, mixing to coat.

Combine & bake: Fold the chocolate mixture into the batter, pour into the prepared loaf pan, and bake for 40-50 minutes, or until a knife inserted in the center comes out clean. *Do not overbake.*
Let cool in the pan for 10 minutes before transferring to a rack. Slice and enjoy!

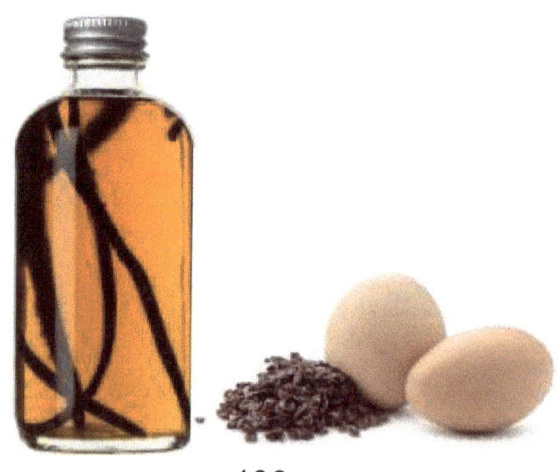

Vocabulary

Antioxidants: Combat free radicals in your body by having unpaired electrons to fight free radicals. Antioxidants carry an extra electron for the free radicals to use because they are missing one. This stops a chain reaction in the body, which would cause inflammation. Antioxidants protect the body against these dangerous molecules by capturing and defusing them, removing them from the cell environment. Antioxidants also offer themselves to be oxidized by the free radicals, but regenerate themselves. Antioxidants also help immensely to repair the damage caused by oxidizing agents. Thus, a healthy level of antioxidants, like vitamin C, vitamin E, and selenium, is essential to prevent chronic inflammatory damage, arrest pre-cancerous changes and slow the so-called aging changes.

Oxidation: The Process of oxidation in the human body damages cell membranes and other structures, including cellular proteins, lipids and DNA. When oxygen is metabolized, it creates 'free radicals' which steal electrons from other molecules, causing damage.

Free Radicals: Usually highly reactive and unstable; missing an electron. As it looks for an electron, it causes a chain reaction, causing oxidation. Antioxidants contain an extra electron and combat free radicals.

Oxidation: Chain reaction caused by the invasion of free radicals, combated by antioxidants.

Phytonutrients (Phytochemicals): Found in plants and have great health benefits to humans.

Glyphosate: First introduced in 1974 under the trade name "Roundup" and has since been marketed under a number of different trade names in hundreds of plant protection products around the world.

Glyphosate: Based herbicides are used to control weeds in a wide range of crops, including cereals, oilseed rape, field beans, sunflowers, grain maize, sugar beet and grassland. Used in genetically modified organisms.

Flavonoids: are plant-based compounds with powerful antioxidant properties found in many fruits and vegetables like blueberries and grapes.

Genetically Modified Organism (GMO): Organisms that have been created through the application of transgenic, gene-splicing techniques that are part of biotechnology. They are foods produced from organisms that have had changes introduced into their dna using the

134

methods of genetic engineering.

Genetically Engineered (GEO): Altered with inserted genetic material to exhibit traits that repel pests or withstand the application of herbicides and round-up. Once G E products are on the market, no labeling is required. This means that U.S. consumers blindly eat and drink **GE** ingredients every day and are not given the knowledge or choice to do otherwise.

Metabolic Syndrome: Is a cluster of conditions — increased blood pressure, high blood sugar, excess body fat around the waist, and abnormal cholesterol or triglyceride levels that occur together, increasing your risk of heart disease, stroke and diabetes.

Excitotoxins: Are substances, usually amino acids, that stimulate taste receptors on the tongue. Not preservatives and with no nutritional value, excitotoxins are nothing other than "chemicals added to foods to make them tastier.

MSG: Monosodium glutamate is an excitotoxin, which means it overexcites your cells to the point of damage or death. msg is more than just a seasoning like salt and pepper; it actually enhances the flavor of foods, making processed meats and frozen dinners taste fresher and smell better, salad dressings more tasty, and canned foods less tinny. MSG may affect hormone production in the body.

Gras: Generally recognized as safe.

Polyphenol: A Generic term for the several thousand plant-based molecules that have antioxidant properties. They are also helpful for regulating enzyme function and stimulating cell receptors.

Aspartame: one of the most widely studied sweeteners, but CSP advises steering clear—citing data suggests slightly increased cancer risk in men, and rat studies linking it to leukemia and lymphoma, NutraSweet, Equal, sugar-twin.

Saccharin: About 350 times sweeter than sugar and is used in diet foods and as a packaged (tabletop) sugar substitute. Many studies on rodents have shown that saccharin can cause cancer of the urinary bladder, especially in males and also causes cancer of the uterus, ovaries, skin, blood vessels, and other organs. Additional studies have shown that saccharin increases the potency of other cancer-causing chemicals. And the best epidemiology (human) study, which was conducted by the National Cancer Institute, found that the use of artificial sweeteners (saccharin and cyclamate) is associated with a higher incidence of bladder cancer.

● Sweet'n Low

● Sugar Twin

● Necta Sweet

● Equal Saccharin

Sucralose: It is calorie-free because our bodies don't break it down. The FDA claims that sucralose is 98 percent pure, but what about the other 2 percent? It contains heavy metals like lead, arsenic, triphenylphosphine oxide, methanol, chlorinated disaccharides, and other potentially dangerous substances. • Splenda • Equal

Stevia Leaf Extract (Rebiana): "Natural" High-Potency Sweetener: "Diet," "No-Sugar," "Sugar-Free" and other products, including beverages, packaged sweeteners, and various foods. A composite herb native to South America whose leaves are the source of a noncaloric sweetener. Also called rebiana, stevioside, rebaudioside A, rebaudioside D, etc.; sold under such brand names as Truvia, Pure Via, and sweet leaf.

Caution: Only buy 100% stevia, watch your ingredients

Resveratrol: An antioxidant which causes the body to efficiently detoxify molecules that oxidize other molecules and tissues. It is a phytoalexin, which means it is a protective antibiotic produced in plants under stress, whether due to fungal attack, drought, ultraviolet irradiation, or inflammation. This molecule helps the plants to fight back and maintain health.

Catechins: Found in green tea and in some fruits and veggies, catechins are high in antioxidants.

Leptin: A hormone produced mainly by adipocytes (fat cells) that is involved in the regulation of body fat. Leptin interacts with areas of the brain that control hunger and behavior and signals that the body has had enough to eat.

Leptin Resistance: When someone has too many fat cells, they produce an overabundance of leptin, and it stops working; your brain doesn't get the signal to stop eating because you are resistant to the signal. Now, the hormone ghrelin kicks in.

Ghrelin: An enzyme produced by stomach lining cells that stimulates appetite.

Synthetic: (Of A Substance) Made by chemical synthesis, especially to imitate a natural product.

Natural: Existing in or caused by nature; not made or caused by humankind. .

About Stephany

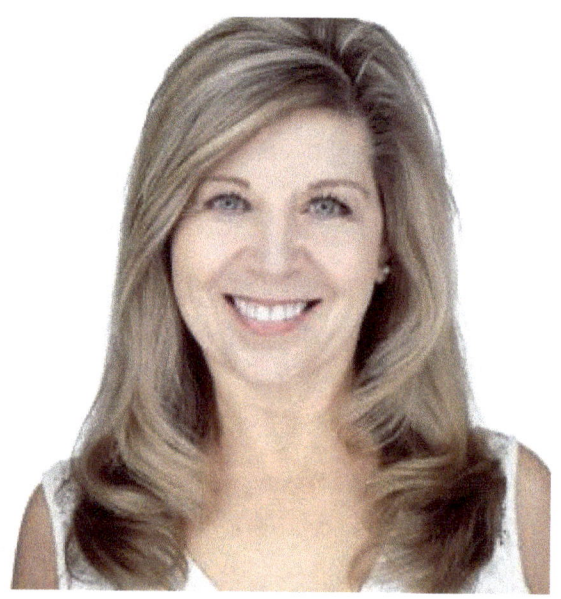

Stephany Baughman began her career as a commercial photographer but transitioned into nutrition after her children were adversely affected by their immunizations, which led her to homeschool them.

This shift led her to explore nutrition deeply, ultimately sparking her passion for health and wellness. She now holds certifications as a Weight Loss Practitioner, Nutritional Advisor, Detox Specialist, Advanced Dietary Supplement Advisor, Nutrition for Cancer Prevention and Longevity, and Menopause Health. Currently, she is studying the Fundamentals of Anatomy, Pathophysiology, and Lifestyle Medicine.

She is the author of several books and cookbooks and has an online course complete with cookbooks, menus, and shopping lists. She still works as a photographer and is a private chef, teacher, and speaker. You can find her course at www.thetastefulplate.com or email her at thetastefulplate@gmail.com

References

American Cancer Society. (n.d.). *What is the best supplement to counteract neuropathy in breast cancer patients?* https://www.google.com/search?q=what+is+the+best+supplement+to+counteract+neuropathy+in+breast+cancer+patients

Bao, T., Basal, C., Seluzicki, C., Li, S. Q., Seidman, A. D., & Mao, J. J. (2014). Long-term chemotherapy-induced peripheral neuropathy among breast cancer survivors: Prevalence, risk factors, and fall risk. *Breast Cancer Research and Treatment, 145*(3), 703-711. https://pmc.ncbi.nlm.nih.gov/articles/PMC4109805

Beth Israel Deaconess Medical Center. (2021). *Eat breakfast.* Living with Cancer Blog. https://www.bidmc.org/about-bidmc/blogs/living-with-cancer/2021/10/eat-breakfast

City of Hope. (2021). *Mushrooms could be a powerful tool against breast cancer.* Retrieved January 2025, from https://www.cityofhope.org/breakthroughs/mushrooms-could-be-a-powerful-tool-against-breast-cancer

Cornell Chronicle. (2004). *Some onions have excellent anti–cancer benefits.* Cornell University. https://news.cornell.edu/stories/2004/10/some-onions-have-excellent-anti-cancer-benefits

Food for Breast Cancer. (n.d.). *Cherries and breast cancer.* https://foodforbreastcancer.com/foods/cherries

Food for Breast Cancer. (n.d.). *Food list.* https://foodforbreastcancer.com/food-list.php

Food for Breast Cancer. (n.d.). *Mushrooms and breast cancer.* Retrieved January 2025, from https://foodforbreastcancer.com/foods/mushrooms

Food for Breast Cancer. (n.d.). *Sugar and breast cancer risk*. Retrieved January 2025, from https://foodforbreastcancer.com/foods/sugar

Healthline. (2019). *Fruits for cancer patients*. https://www.healthline.com/nutrition/fruits-for

-

cancer-

Loma Linda University Health. (2021). *Foods that fight breast cancer*. Retrieved January 2025, from https://news.llu.edu/health-wellness/foods-fight-breast-cancer

MD Anderson Cancer Center. (2021). *3 nutrients cancer survivors should know: Flaxseed, Omega–3s, and Iron*. https://www.mdanderson.org/cancerwise/3-nutrients-cancer-survivors-should-know-flaxseed-omega-3s-iron.h00-159305412.html

National Breast Cancer Foundation. (2020). *5–step ultimate smoothie guide*. Retrieved January 2025, from https://www.nationalbreastcancer.org/blog/5-step-ultimate-smoothie-guide/

OSF HealthCare. (2021). *Cancer–fighting power of tomatoes*. Retrieved January 2025, from https://newsroom.osfhealthcare.org/cancer-fighting-power-of-tomatoes/

Thomson, C. A., Rock, C. L., Thompson, P. A., Caan, B. J., Cussler, E., Flatt, S. W., & Pierce, J. P. (2011). Vegetable intake is associated with reduced breast cancer recurrence in tamoxifen users: A secondary analysis from the Women's Healthy Eating and Living Study. *Breast Cancer Research and Treatment, 125*(2), 519-527. https://doi.org/10.1007/s10549-010-1014-9

www.ingramcontent.com/pod-product-compliance
Lightning Source LLC
Chambersburg PA
CBHW041116120626

46547CB00019B/2733